NOBODY KNOWS THE TROUBLE I'VE SEEN

THE
EMOTIONAL
LIVES OF
BLACK
WOMEN

Praise for *Nobody Knows the Trouble I've Seen*

"Excellent debut . . . This thorough analysis effectively pulls back the curtain on the emotional and health barriers Black women face to suggest practical strategies for change."

—*Publishers Weekly*

"Provides both practical and clinical advice with an emphasis on improving Black women's emotional and physical health through trauma resolution, exercise, mindfulness, support systems, self-compassion, setting boundaries, and seeking joy."

—New York Journal of Books

"Black women give and give and give to the point of emotional exhaustion. *Nobody Knows the Trouble I've Seen* lets us know how to break this unhealthy cycle by learning self-forgiveness, which through God's help, leads to self-love and the power to say, 'No, I come first in my life.'" —Mary J. Blige

"Through a blend of irrefutable scientific data and deeply moving personal narratives, Inger Burnett-Zeigler's *Nobody Knows the Trouble I've Seen* takes an unflinching look at the sources of Black women's pain and explodes the myth that our strength comes without sacrifice. This book invites us to be our whole, authentic selves—capable, yes, but also vulnerable and deserving of love and care. *Nobody Knows the Trouble I've Seen* is an offering, an affirmation, a balm, and a road map to transformation and real healing—a gift to Black women everywhere."

—Natalie Baszile, author of *Queen Sugar* and *We Are Each Other's Harvest: Celebrating African American Farmers, Land, and Legacy*

"Patience, courage, and perseverance are required in taking good care of yourself. You are worthy. You are important. Your song is part of a great symphony! *Nobody Knows the Trouble I've Seen* will help you find your instrument and melody."

—Jenifer Lewis, author of *The Mother of Black Hollywood*

"'Listen to Black women' and 'Black Girl Magic' are common phrases these days. Inger Burnett-Zeigler reveals what is unsaid about the Strong Black Woman—she needs to tend to her own individual health. This book is affirming and full of lessons."

—Natalie Y. Moore, author of *The South Side: A Portrait of Chicago and American Segregation*

"*Nobody Knows the Trouble I've Seen* speaks to the stress and trauma that many Black women have experienced in various aspects of their lives. Dr. Burnett-Zeigler has written an essential guidebook for Black women to investigate what healing looks like and finally feel seen." —Minda Harts, author of *Right Within*

NOBODY KNOWS THE TROUBLE I'VE SEEN

INGER BURNETT-ZEIGLER, PhD

AMISTAD
— 35 —

An Imprint of HarperCollinsPublishers

HarperCollins books may be purchased for educational, business, or sales promotional use. For information, please email the Special Markets Department at SPsales@harpercollins.com.

FIRST HARPERCOLLINS PAPERBACK EDITION PUBLISHED IN 2022

Designed by THE COSMIC LION

Library of Congress Cataloging-in-Publication Data is available upon request.

ISBN 978-0-06-295983-6

22 23 24 25 26 LSC 10 9 8 7 6 5 4 3 2 1

To my mom,
for your strength and vulnerability,
lifetime of sacrifice,
and abundant love.

"Usually when people talk about the 'strength' of black women they are referring to the way in which they perceive black women coping with oppression. They ignore the reality that to be strong in the face of oppression is not the same as overcoming oppression, that endurance is not to be confused with transformation."

bell hooks, *ain't i a woman*

Contents

VULNERABILITY

HEALING

NOBODY KNOWS THE TROUBLE I'VE SEEN

Introduction

Everywhere that we turn, we're surrounded by beautiful, intelligent, strong Black women. I'm sure that you can name many in your own life. In fact, you're probably one of them. Today's strong Black women are grinding at work and climbing professional ladders, at every event, hair laid, nails done, dressed to perfection and nowhere is a trace of trouble to be found. They are sitting next to you at church, volunteering at community events, and at your book or wine club. They are doing whatever they need to do to take care of their children and extended family, with or without the help of a partner. They are working multiple jobs, trying to make it in a system designed to prevent them from getting ahead. Strong Black women are not just the backbone of society, they are its breath and its heartbeat.

The strong Black woman can be seen on big and small screens or one click away on social media. Political leaders like Shirley Chisholm, Auntie Maxine, and Michelle Obama; literary icons like Gwendolyn Brooks, Octavia Butler, and Toni Morrison; athletic champions like Althea Gibson and Serena Williams; dynamic actresses like Cicely Tyson, Angela Bassett, and Regina King; and TV moms like Florida Evans and Clair Huxtable. Crooners who *sang* such as Aretha Franklin, Nina Simone, and Mary J. Blige. And, representing business leaders, Ursula M. Burns, Debra Lee, and Mellody Hobson. They are also those in our own families whose names may be lesser known, like my grandmother and mother, my first strong Black women examples; the women who mentor me at work; and, of course, my girlfriends.

From a distance, strong Black women seem invincible. Everything they set out to accomplish, they achieve. They bounce back stronger from whatever threatens to get in their way. Their head is always held up high, with style and a smile. If you step out of line and need to be put back in your place, they can do that too. Above all, they never forget to give praise and honor to God for all that he has done for them. We look up to these women as our role models and for inspiration. Their strength makes us believe that the possibilities available to us are limitless.

But, as strong Black women, you know best that it isn't always easy to be strong. The world is out here testing us every day, be it at home, work, or just walking down the street. My grandmother taught my mother, and my mother taught me, to deal with hurt, disappointment, and loss by wiping my tears away, keeping my head up and keeping going. *It ain't the first time you've been hurt and it won't be the last*, she would say. My mother reminded me early and often, *Life ain't fair, so don't expect it to be.*

Society puts pressure on us to be everything to everybody—to be superwomen—and we accept the charge. We are constantly pouring out and rarely allow ourselves to receive the care we so urgently need. We fight tooth and nail to defy the negative expectations people have of us and to prove our worth. And yet, it seems like it's never enough.

In spite of our difficult circumstances, Black women are masters at maintaining a cool indifference and presenting ourselves as having it all together. As soon as we step out of the house, we put our game face on—our mask. This mask is our protection from all of the historical trauma and societal ills—racism, sexism, victimization—that weigh us down. It tries to keep the outside hurt from getting in and the inside hurt from getting out.

Often the mask is a façade and doesn't really reflect what we've been through or how we're feeling. Although we generally accept the label of strong Black woman with pride, on the other side of the mask are stress, anxiety, and depression that lead to unhealthy behaviors such as emotional eating, poor sleep, and neglecting self-care. The mask allows us to show only a fraction of our true selves to the world. We wear it as a way of coping with our pain. It's our survival tactic. But is it really serving us? I don't think so. In fact, I believe the strong Black woman mask is preventing us from being our authentic and abundant selves.

When all forms of suffering are considered, it's hard to find a Black woman who hasn't experienced some form of trauma. Yet if you don't look closely, or ask the right questions, you would look right past them. Black women have been pushing through and going through the motions for so long that suffering has become the norm. Far too often we have coped with our pain by turning away from it, avoiding or denying it rather than looking at it closely and handling it tenderly.

Nobody Knows the Trouble I've Seen is about strong Black women, the unknown suffering that is intimately embedded in their strength. It is a guidebook for healing. In this book I will show you how to move past the façade of the strong Black woman and embrace who you really are—warm and supportive, audacious, and joyous.

The woman who is "too strong" lives a life in which she doesn't acknowledge all of the emotions that are a part of a normal human experience. The woman who is "too vulnerable" may be less equipped to cope in today's society, where systematic oppression and racial and gender discrimination are rampant. Here, I will outline how Black women can create a healthy balance between strength and vulnerability.

Long before I ever started trying to understand the circumstances that shape the lives of others, I observed and analyzed what was happening within my own household. Early on I realized that my mother and grandmother were only revealing a fraction of themselves to the outside world. They made it clear that not all things are granted permission to be openly discussed, and emotions are complex and at times may feel contradictory. By middle school I'd determined that my family was dysfunctional and suggested to my parents that we go to therapy, a novel idea for a little Black girl living on the South Side of Chicago. I wanted to fix us. I wanted our family to be *normal*.

My mother's response was to ignore it. *What do you think we need therapy for?* she asked with genuine confusion. My dad chuckled with amusement, attempting to assure me, *We're fine.* And, they both went on: *We aren't the kind of people who go to therapy. This was some mess that you must have picked up from the white kids at school.* They were right.

I attended a liberal and racially diverse elementary school. When the kids at my school had a problem, the entire family sat around in a circle and talked to a kind and understanding person who listened carefully and helped them to work it out. At least that's how I imagined it to be. Those white kids seemed happy and well adjusted.

Instead of talking about our problems, I learned how to pretend that everything was normal and to keep my thoughts and feelings to myself. This behavior worked temporarily, until eventually all of the emotions that I had been suppressing came rising to the surface. It's also the reason I decided to write *Nobody Knows the Trouble I've Seen*, because I know that suppressing how you feel doesn't make the feelings, or the problems, go away.

As a clinical psychologist, I bring together a lifetime of observing, listening to, and learning from strong Black women, decades of scholarly research that has been conducted on their mental and physical health, and experience providing mental health treatment. I also offer you my lived experiences as a Black woman who has struggled with depression and anxiety.

In the pages to come it is my intention to honor and celebrate the strong Black woman, and also help us to take the necessary steps to be emotionally and physically well—as the two are intricately entwined. Every strong Black woman holds an untold story, and here we'll begin to reveal the challenges that we face and learn wellness practices to build a community of authentically strong women from the inside out. I invite you to open your heart and mind. I invite you to use your voice, be heard, and ask for what we need from our partners, our managers, and our children. I invite you to release the suffering that you've been holding onto for so long. In this way we will continue to make impactful contributions to the world, and in our own lives, by abandoning self-defeating behaviors.

Throughout the book, I unearth the many issues we as Black women deal with daily. We will explore how trauma and adversity have led to deep emotional pain that has shaped our lives. For instance, I discuss the stress brought on from work and financial issues and from being regularly confronted by racism and discrimination. I share with you stories about childhood sexual abuse, domestic violence, relationship baggage, pregnancy trauma, absentee fathers, and mother-child separation. This work challenges the tradition of secret keeping in our community and its relationship to intergenerational patterns and cycles that perpetuate suffering. It also shows you how to recognize mental health challenges and offers strategies for healing.

Nobody Knows the Trouble I've Seen features many different women. Along the way you will get to know my beloved grandmother and mother and the ways that their life experiences have impacted me. I will show you how they passed down their strength, and, unknowingly, generational trauma, like your grandmothers and mothers may have inadvertently done with you. My clients have also graciously allowed me to tell their stories. But I have changed their names to protect their privacy, and I did the same for friends who were willing to participate.

In therapy, my clients and I explore what lies beneath the mask of strength. This is usually an unfamiliar space, because talking about our problems to strangers is not something we as Black women typically do. But if you have come to this book, you might be willing to try something new to help you with all that you have been holding onto. Don't be afraid of what might happen if you unearth a buried part of yourself. I invite you to approach the pain that for years has been avoided and denied. You no longer have to pretend that you're "fine."

Research has shown that people who have experienced trauma are more vulnerable to a wide range of challenges, such as academic and behavioral problems in childhood; high-risk pregnancy; negative birth outcomes (i.e., premature birth); poor physical health outcomes like higher rates of obesity, diabetes, and cardiovascular disease; and poor mental health outcomes like stress, anxiety, depression, and suicidal thoughts. When the traumatic histories of Black women are compounded with day-to-day acute and chronic stress, the outcomes can be detrimental.

At the start of therapy women are generally unaware of how trauma and chronic stress have impacted their emotions, behavior, and ability to function day to day. But they want something to ease their sadness and worry. Often they feel lost and are looking for insight and hope. My clients share things with me that no one else in their life knows, entrusting me with the most vulnerable parts of themselves. They discover their own wants and needs after years of taking care of everyone else and neglecting themselves. I help them to understand the impact that trauma has had on their lives and to transition from feeling stuck in suffering to being empowered to take steps toward healing. I underscore the importance of being mindfully aware of your own thoughts, feelings, and behaviors; identifying sources of stress; confronting problems head on; and embracing support. I encourage women to let go of ideals and expectations, and create space for their authentic selves while giving permission to take care of themselves. It is my goal that our work together of peeling back the accumulated layers of suffering helps them to find their true selves, where their full power and potential lie.

Through the examples in this book, I will show you how these women were able to move from the antiquated model of being strong, which requires denying and suppressing feelings, to being strong in a way that allowed them to acknowledge their suffering, cope in healthier ways, and heal. You may find that you relate to some of the women. As you go through the pages, I invite you to reflect on your own life experiences. It is my hope that through these stories, you will be able to take a closer look at the things that have been weighing you down and holding you back and let them go. I will give you a new framework within which to compassionately honor all parts of yourself. I hope that this book will be the beginning of the healing process for you.

Nobody Knows the Trouble I've Seen is about truly seeing strong Black women in our fullness and the beauty within both our strength and our vulnerability. I want us to redefine what it means to be strong, embrace the opportunity for vulnerability, and let go of the feelings of shame that may come up in the process. Ultimately, my desire is that this book will give women the power to make new choices for what they want for themselves and to live longer, healthier lives.

"Freeing yourself was one thing, claiming ownership of that freed self was another."

TONI MORRISON, *Beloved*

STRENGTH

We wear the mask that grins and lies.
It shades our cheeks and hides our eyes.
This debt we pay to human guile
With torn and bleeding hearts . . .
We smile and mouth the myriad subtleties.
Why should the world think otherwise
In counting all our tears and sighs.
Nay let them only see us while
We wear the mask.

MAYA ANGELOU, *We Wear the Mask*

I Am a Strong Black Woman

If you want to get something done, "ask a Black woman" is a saying that goes way back in our community. And the world shows us nearly every day how true this is. Want to change a historically red state to blue, ask Stacey Abrams. Want to put a man on the moon, ask Katherine Johnson. Want to begin to solve the food insecurity issues, ask Leah Penniman. From an early age, little Black girls, who eventually grow up to be strong Black women, are taught how to be tough and take care of business—not out of choice, but necessity. Our mothers know that strength will be required for us to survive and make it in the world, so we have to wipe our tears aside and keep it moving.

Strong Black women role models teach us how to function in the world. We listen to them—what is said, and what is left unsaid. We watch closely how they handle life's challenges. We take in not only their strength, but also their style, rhythm, and bellowing laughter. When we see other women killing it, doing the thing, we revel in their success, and it lifts the whole of us. We know that when one of us pushes through, she leaves a path for more to follow. We are proud to be a part of this sisterhood of beauty, intelligence, and *magic*. Being strong has become so deeply engrained in us that we don't know any other way to be.

Being a strong Black woman has historically been the essence of Black femininity. For decades, this prototype has provided the blueprint for how to appropriately perform our race-gender identity.[1] In terms of role expectations, a strong Black woman is a provider, caretaker, and homemaker. Whether it's because she chooses to do so or is required to do so as a single parent or head of household, she is able to independently provide for herself and her family. Miraculously, she succeeds despite having minimal resources. She can handle everything on her own; she doesn't *need* anyone for anything. Her independence allows her to maintain a sense of control over herself and her circumstances.

A strong Black woman is ambitious, determined to be *the best*, and she understands that she will have to work harder in every aspect of her life in order to prove her value. She may be the first in her family to attain certain educational and professional achievements, such as graduating from college, obtaining an advanced degree, or being in a position of management. She is intent on discrediting the negative views that society has about Black women as hypersexual, lazy underachievers and failures who are looking for a handout.

The strong Black woman has been trained to put the needs of others—especially family—ahead of her own. This can mean sacrificing personal hopes, dreams, aspirations, and especially time for self-care, in order to take care of children, as mothers often do. As she achieves career success, the strong Black woman may feel responsible for helping people in her family and community, which sometimes can lead to a sense of pride, purpose, and value and other times can leave her feeling worn down, stressed, and overwhelmed. She may develop a *savior complex*, whereby she believes that she's the only one around who can get things done—and get them done right. She becomes attached to her role as "the strong one" or "the fixer." It feels good to her to know that she is needed. If she doesn't take care of things, nobody will.

Despite being stretched thin, she has difficulty setting boundaries and saying *No*, sometimes out of guilt for being the one who made it and not wanting to be perceived as "too" good. She feels a sense of indebtedness to her ancestors and future generations to give everything that she has. In this way, the strong Black woman can become a martyr, or as Zora Neale Hurston described it in her 1937 novel, *Their Eyes Were Watching God*, "de mule uh de world," by carrying a load so heavy that she sacrifices her individual health for the good of the whole.

Even with the weight that she shoulders, the strong Black woman holds her head up high, appears confident and proud. Her pride is reflected in her purposeful walk, assertive voice, and deliberate actions. She is a leader in her family, church, and community. Her belief in God, who gives her strength and makes all things possible, is her anchor. She works hard to preserve her image of strength for the sake of those who depend on and look up to her. In the face of adversity, she is resilient and never loses hope.

A problem comes up, however, when we Black women believe that we should appear strong even when we don't feel strong. We hide the aspects of ourselves that we think are inconsistent with strength in order to maintain our respectable, strong Black woman standing.

We have accepted the pretense that being strong means not acknowledging our true feelings and keeping things inside. It's the stern or expressionless face that is often misperceived as being mean, hard, or angry. The emotions of sadness, fear, and worry are rarely revealed because we are concerned that they might be labeled soft or weak. The strong Black woman worries that if people know that she has such feelings, they will think that she is a failure or, worse, crazy. The mismatch between the reality of our feelings and the façade of strength eats away at us over time and can eventually reveal itself as mental distress and physical illness.

In the mind of a strong Black woman, vulnerability puts her at greater risk for being hurt or taken advantage of, so she keeps her defenses up. It is hard for her to trust people. The idea of letting go of control by sharing her most private thoughts and feelings, or having to depend on someone else, is intolerable. Besides, she doesn't want to inconvenience or burden anyone else with her problems because they've got problems of their own. We believe it's up to the strong Black woman to protect and take care of herself, because surely nobody else will.

The prototype strong Black woman was born of the systematic and institutional racism, sexism, and oppression that has disenfranchised Black women and their families for centuries. A history of disappointment, mistreatment, or abuse has contributed to and maintained the strong Black woman legacy. Many Black women have been so repeatedly and systematically let down by people in their families, communities, and institutions that they have become resigned to their pain as a companion of life. This coping style was developed as a survival mechanism, but it has been maintained as a cultural standard and continues to bear incredible costs.

Lessons on how to be a strong Black woman have been passed down for generations from grandmothers, mothers, aunts, and sisters through dialogue, modeling, and conditioning. These role models have preached the importance of being able to protect and care for ourselves, while keeping secret their personal stories of

struggle and suppressing their inner emotions. There is an unspoken sentiment that if our foremothers survived the brutal and dehumanizing conditions of slavery, we—the generations of women
who follow them—should be able to handle anything. But what we
don't recognize is that trauma experienced by past generations is
cumulative and it shows up in us.

We've come to believe that suffering is just a part of life and
living—Black women's living. For us, a life without suffering is an
unfamiliar indulgence. To be strong and to overcome in the face of
struggle can become such an inherent part of what it means to be
a Black woman that we have difficulty evaluating ourselves by any
other metric.

My grandmother was one of my first examples of a strong
Black woman. She left her man and Montgomery, Alabama, in
1951 and headed north as a single mother along with millions of
other Black people during the second wave of the Great Migration
in pursuit of better employment opportunities, and perhaps also a
new suitor. At that time, fewer than 20 percent of Black families
had a female head of household with no husband present.[2] When
she arrived in Chicago in 1954, after making a pit stop in Pennsylvania, she and my mother lived in a one-bedroom apartment
on the West Side in the Jane Addams Homes. The public housing
complex was initially built for impoverished Italian and Russian-
Jewish residents. They moved out of the neighborhood as Black
families were beginning to trickle in, along with several notorious
street gangs.

Despite the welfare laws that prohibited Grandma from working, she held a job as a seamstress. She made curtains during the
day and attended Crane Junior College at night. Assured that her
fate would ultimately turn, she rolled the dice on herself and played

her numbers in the policy game—the underground lottery in the neighborhood. Her younger sisters, who remained in their distressed marriages, sent money to help fill in the financial gaps of the husband she'd left behind. But my grandmother's thorny temperament ensured that they remained on the outskirts of her and my mother's lives and kept them isolated and without the emotional support that they didn't know they needed.

Grandma never rested in "good enough." With every accomplishment, the lust for the sufficiency of validation dwindled only slightly. For more than thirty years, she worked as an unemployment counselor at the State of Illinois Department of Labor. When I went to work with her as a little girl, I imagined that I, too, had an important job helping people—answering the phone and writing memos that would ultimately change the course of someone's life. The constant flow of other people not having enough kept my grandmother moving forward. She quietly repaid her debts to the system that had helped her to claw her way out of poverty. Yet she could never afford to let down her defenses.

Eventually, when she was more than fifty years old, Grandma moved out of public housing and returned to school through a program offered by her employer to earn her bachelor's degree at Roosevelt University. At that time only 8 percent of Black women in the United States had a college education.[3] In the early 1970s, when predatory lending, redlining, and restrictive covenants were rampant in Chicago, she purchased a ranch house facing the train tracks in the previously Dutch community of Roseland. White flight was at its peak as Black folks rapidly began to occupy the neighborhood.

With every visit I made to Grandma's house, she planted the seeds of my self-worth and willed to me her expectations for greatness. They were steeped in the Lipton's lemon tea that we sweetened with packs of Equal and sipped out of pink porcelain teacups. We drank and held our pinkies out while speaking in fake British accents. She and I sat in perfect manner in her ornate wooden dining room chairs, which swallowed my petite frame and left my feet dangling beneath the table. As we delicately placed the teacups down on the saucers, we pursed our lips together and fluttered our eyelids, mimicking the air that we imagined rich and important people had. "Be still and stop kicking," Grandma said, teaching me how to be proper and dignified.

Grandma's hope for me was interlaced between her fingers as she kneeled down on the floor with me next to the bed as I said my prayers—*Now I lay me down to sleep, I pray the Lord my soul to keep, and if I die before I wake, I pray the Lord my soul to take*—being sure to ask God to bless Grandma, Mommy, and Daddy. In the morning she sent me home with a promise for prosperity folded in greeting cards that held an *Our Daily Bread* devotional booklet and twenty crisp dollar bills that she slid to me behind my mother's back. "A third for you, a third for tithes, and a third for your piggy bank and one day you'll be rich like Grandma," she said.

For many of us, our grandmother sets the precedent that we strive to follow. When you need something, be it a few extra dollars, a place to stay, or just some solid advice, she's the one you go to. She may not have much, but whatever she does have, she offers it to you freely. She's a truth-teller who doesn't mince words or spare feelings. She shows her love through her fierce loyalty to her family, steadfast nature, good cooking, and faithful prayers. The well of her wisdom runs deep. She's tough, but beneath her tough exterior, she has stories to tell.

But while my grandmother taught me how to be strong, I was

left to my own devices to figure out how to cope with the difficult emotions of anxiety, depression, and even suicidal thoughts that started to creep in by adolescence. As I struggled to understand my "nontraditional" family, and sought out a sense of belonging and acceptance, I flailed in a pool of erratic emotions that I didn't understand. It wasn't until I found myself in an unhealthy intimate relationship in my twenties that I finally sought out therapy.

With the help of therapy, my faith in God, and a mindfulness meditation and yoga practice—and the support of a community of amazing, strong Black women—I slowly stopped feeling so depressed, anxious, damaged, and unsure of myself. I learned how to cope with the low moods and bouts of worry that inevitably come from time to time. When I feel down, I am able to acknowledge and hold space for that emotion, rather than ignore it or push it aside. When I feel anxious, I identify the worry, redirect my attention to things I can control, and let go of the rest. I affirm my needs, have firm and clear boundaries, practice gratitude, and take plenty of guilt-free time for rest and pleasure. But even with all of that, I can still be a strong Black woman.

As a clinical psychologist, I help Black women examine the parts of the strong Black woman prototype that continue to serve us—such as compassion, loving care for others, community orientation, determination, resilience, self-assuredness, faith in God, joyfulness—while leaving behind the parts that no longer serve us: suppressing emotion, denying our needs, being reluctant to set boundaries and say *No*, overworking, and not asking for help. When we grab hold of our strengths and release our difficulties and challenges, we are well-positioned to start the healing journey.

Along this journey I help my clients identify their vulnerabilities (which are often rooted in past trauma), understand their current needs in service of mental wellness and healthy relationships, and relearn what it means to take care of themselves. I ask clients to consider the at-times-hard-to-believe possibility that there is space to take care of themselves AND others, and that caring for others doesn't have to mean deprioritizing or sacrificing the self.

This is an ongoing process of learning that self-care is not selfish, boundaries are necessary, and rest is required for rejuvenation. It is by filling our own cup that we have a wealth of abundance from which we can give to others. It is by caring for ourselves that we are able to tap in to our divine light and let that energy resonate widely.

Together, my clients and I reshape previously written narratives that discount their inherent worth, challenge expectations about who they *should* be and what they *should* do, and release the intentions that they want to manifest in the future. It is high time for us as Black women to resist the subjugation to martyrdom and redefine strength in a way that includes being strong enough to take care of ourselves and chart the course of our own destinies.

This means being strong enough to say "I too have feelings," "I too am important," and "My needs and wants also matter." We must stop exhausting ourselves by trying to perform some idealized role of how we *should* be or what a "real" strong Black woman looks like. We don't have to accept the role of provider or selfless caregiver just because it has been thrust upon us. Although we are part of a community, we are also whole individuals, and our existence does not have to be solely defined by what we do for others.

Far too often we falsely believe that we don't have any choice in how we go through life, but we do. It is time for us as Black women to take control of our own lives, rather than letting the world, and tradition and expectation, direct our lives for us. We can choose the roles that we want to take on and carry them out in our own way. We don't have to continue to do things the way that they have always been done. We can break the cycle. Our health depends on our making a grand change.

Let me remind you that although you may have become accustomed to suffering, inside of you lies the capacity for peace and contentment. The lightness and freedom of joy is indeed possible. You have the power to tap in to this ever-flowing stream, revel in it, and share it with everyone you meet. Your healing and discovery of inner peace break the cycle of suffering not just for you, but also for those who are in this time with you and those who will come after you.

TWO

On My Last Nerve

You don't have to look too far to see a Black woman shining in the workplace. This is also the place where we experience the most obstacles. For example, if you work for yourself, you are typically barred access to crucial resources such as investment capital. If you work for corporate America, you deal with regular racial insensitivities and microaggressions like not being seen, heard, or adequately rewarded for your contributions and accomplishments. And if you happen to be employed in a primarily Black space of business, you may have to deal with "crabs in a barrel" mentalities.

In short, work and life issues come with more than their fair share of stress. According to the 2010 *Stress in America* survey published by the American Psychological Association, money, work, family responsibilities, personal health, family health, and the economy are the most common sources of stress. Many Black women have added stress related to trauma, poverty, racism, sexism, and discrimination.[1]

In an informal social media poll that I conducted among Black women in my network, participants reported the following stressors:

- Making and saving money
- Experiencing microaggressions at work—everyday, subtle, intentional and sometimes unintentional interactions or behaviors that communicate racism and discrimination
- Being the only Black woman, or one of few, in the workplace
- Being the first in the family to "make it"
- Dealing with white privilege
- Experiencing imposter syndrome (more on this below)
- Feeling under a microscope
- Being afraid of disappointing themselves or others
- Feeling not good enough
- Having to provide for and take care of children
- Being a single parent
- Feeling concerned about the safety of their Black sons
- Feeling unsafe
- Trying to be "superwoman" as a wife or partner, mother, and employee
- Balancing work and life
- Having to "save the day" for struggling family members by paying bills, loaning money, providing bail money, and solving problems
- Having to care for other family members, such as aging parents
- Planning for the future
- Just trying to live as a Black person

This list makes clear the toll that being a provider and caretaker in a racist and sexist society takes on Black women's mental health and well-being.

The importance of the Black woman's role in the labor market was established during slavery in the eighteenth and nineteenth centuries and with sharecropping in the nineteenth and twentieth centuries.[2] As providers, we participate in the labor force at higher rates than white women, yet still, at all educational levels, we are overrepresented in lower-paying jobs that have little security, few benefits, and few opportunities for advancement. Because of institutional racism, Black men do not make as much as their white counterparts, so Black women are left to take on more of a family's financial burden or become a sole breadwinner.[3] More than 80 percent of Black mothers are either the sole earner or earn at least 40 percent of the income in their households. Three-quarters of Black women who are breadwinners are doing so alone.[4]

A 2017 piece by the National Center for Education Statistics reported that Black women are earning more college degrees than any other racial/ethnic group;[5] however, college-educated Black women still earn less than white women who are not college educated. Despite being the most educated group, Black women make up only 8 percent of the corporate workforce and 2 percent of senior executives, which, in addition to its financial implications, contributes to social isolation and feelings of loneliness.[6]

In professional positions, Black women are often held to a higher standard of performance. We are asked to do more and put in more hours, and sometimes asked to cover for co-workers who are not up to speed, yet somehow it seems that we can never get ahead. We do extra service work, such as planning professional-development or team-building activities, leading special-interest groups for women or African Americans, such as Diversity and Inclusion programming; or mentoring junior staff. All these activities are time and labor intensive, but we get little reward for our involvement, and they do not count toward our advancement.

The devaluation of our contributions can leave us feeling demoralized. Although we take on the responsibility to mentor and lift up younger women, especially Black women, we usually have few mentors or sponsors of our own to help us navigate the politics of the workplace. We're expected to always say *Yes!* and appear friendly and eager, and if we don't, we risk being labeled "angry" or "not a team player," and we're left feeling alienated. We work overtime trying to network, prove that we belong, and learn the rules of a game that we are not meant to know, while never really feeling like we fit in. We are exhausted by *always* having to be "on." In the mostly white spaces in which we work, we have little room for error. With every step that we take, the bar moves farther away, and our self-assuredness disintegrates.

Although the majority of Black women are breadwinners, Black female unemployment is higher than the rate for women from other racial/ethnic groups and higher than the rate for men from all racial/ethnic groups (except for Black men: 8.9 percent for Black women compared with 10.3 percent for Black men). Black women experience poverty at higher rates than Black men and women from all other racial/ethnic groups. A quarter of Black women in the United States live in poverty, compared with 10.8 percent of white women.[7]

Poverty-related stress comes with worry about being able to cover basic needs such as food, housing, and childcare; living in a safe neighborhood; taking public transportation; having a reliable car; and having the ability to pay for an emergency should one arise. But being in a place of lack is not always because you did something wrong. Surely, there are more people living paycheck to paycheck, struggling to make ends meet, than there are with disposable income. This scenario is not likely to change anytime soon, as the COVID pandemic has made economic stability even more challenging for many.

Women who are living in poverty can feel like they are one disaster away from losing everything. If the furnace breaks, the car needs work, or one of the kids has a big medical bill, there won't be enough money to cover it. Not to mention the pressure that comes from trying to scrape up enough money to do something nice once in awhile, such as host a baby shower, take a vacation, or save enough money for a college fund.

On the other hand, when we do "make it" and get the big salaries, the persistent feeling of "not enoughness" can impact our financial health. In order to fill the void that is created by a world that constantly tells us we are lacking something as a Black woman, we can find ourselves overcompensating with *things*—expensive cars, designer purses, lavish vacations—that we may think serve as external markers of worth. Whether we're doing it for the gram or trying to keep up with the Joneses, we buy things that we don't need and perhaps can't afford just to prove *I am somebody*. However, the validation that is achieved from acquiring things lasts for only a moment. Before we know it, we are looking for something else to fill the void.

Instead, we have to remind ourselves that with or without the accoutrement, we shine the brightest from the inside out. Emotionally driven spending behaviors can prevent us from growing our wealth for the next generation and keep us one bad day away from being back in poverty again.

Poverty, racism, and discrimination are inextricably linked. Housing segregation due to racism can lead to fewer opportunities for high-quality education through attending good schools, leaving us with fewer employment opportunities. Even when we secure a job, we are regularly underemployed, meaning holding a position for which we are overqualified. Black men have disproportionately higher rates of involvement with the criminal justice system, which not only breaks apart our families and erodes our morale, but also can leave more women to be the sole earners in their households. When we face mental and physical illnesses, they are more disabling because we have less access to high-quality health care. In turn, we are less able to remain productive and engaged in the workforce and to care for our families.

To be sure, racism and discrimination impact all Black people regardless of where they fall on the socioeconomic spectrum. More than 70 percent of Black adults report experiencing day-to-day discrimination, such as being treated with less courtesy or respect, being treated as if they are not smart, or receiving poor service; and more than 60 percent of Black adults say that their lives are at least a little harder because of discrimination.[8] These instances can range from being racially profiled by police, being presumed to be in an administrative support position rather than one of leadership, being paid less than less-experienced colleagues, being denied a job or promotion, and being dismissed by a healthcare provider— such as the time I asked my ob/gyn about freezing my eggs, and her response was, "Can you even afford that option?" Or when I walk into a high-end retail store, with uncombed hair, wearing yoga pants, looking like every other white girl in the neighborhood, and no one asks me if I need help.

While we're trying to come up, racism continuously has its foot on our necks. Racism is associated with increased work-related stress and lower job satisfaction. We can find ourselves feeling keyed up and on edge when we have a racist encounter and we try to control our reactions and say and do the "right" thing. *Microaggressions* can be particularly insidious—such as when a co-worker questions how your parents afforded to send you to private school, or asks whether you heard gunshots in your neighborhood when you were growing up on the South Side of Chicago, or says that you're different than those *other* Black people, or is surprised at the quality of your work, or believes that it is your responsibility to mentor *all* of the Black student interns because you will "understand" and "relate to" them better. It can feel impossible to find the right words to address such microaggressions head-on while maintaining decorum. We question ourselves and wonder whether we are perceiving the interaction accurately. *Did he just say what I think he said?* we ask ourselves. *Am I the one who's crazy?* No, you're not the one who's crazy. An estimated 25 percent of Black women report experiencing microaggressions at least monthly; 10 percent report experiencing them weekly or multiple times per week.[9] These microaggressions chip away at our mental health like a million tiny little cuts.

In majority-white schools and workplaces, we can become hyperaware of our mere existence and others' response to it. We battle with *imposter syndrome*—feelings of self-doubt and inadequacy despite external evidence of accomplishment and success. Without a doubt, imposter syndrome is not all in our heads but is bred by racist and sexist systems that tell us that we are inadequate. For instance, one Black woman had exceeded performance expectations for three straight years in her white-dominated industry. When she asked her boss for a promotion, her boss started to tell the employee about her own career trajectory, which did not include a college degree. Then the boss went on to explain to the college-educated employee why she was not qualified. To cope with feeling like an

imposter, we tend to cling to excessively high standards and perfec-
tionistic ideals. We place incredible pressure on ourselves to meet
these standards, which contributes to stress and anxiety, and our
self-worth becomes contingent on achieving.

If we don't achieve a goal that we're aiming for—the degree,
the job, the promotion, the money, the material things—again,
we feel shame and question whether we are good enough. If we do
achieve the goal, we may minimize our accomplishments as being
due to luck or people mistakenly thinking that we're better than we
really are. Even with positive feedback, we can be suspicious and
nontrusting of how we are being evaluated behind closed doors
and have an enduring sense of not belonging. This fear of being a
fraud can prevent us from going after new opportunities or putting
ourselves out there and being visible rather than shrinking into the
background.

In the workplace, we also wrestle with *stereotype threat*—the
fear of confirming negative stereotypes associated with our race/
gender group, such as being "ghetto," angry, lazy, or not smart. If
we wear our hair in braids to the office, eat fried chicken for lunch,
admit to listening to ratchet music or watching trash reality TV,
or use our at-home intonation, we fear that we will be inaccurately
summed up and reduced to a cliché by our peers. We carry the
weight of representing well not only for ourselves, but our entire
community. In an attempt to conform, appear socially acceptable
by mainstream standards, and control how others perceive us, we
may slip into playing *respectability politics*, which means quieting
our voices and hiding parts of ourselves and our culture. However,
a 2013 study that colleagues and I conducted found that Black
people who had a *stronger* ethnic identity—sense of pride, belonging, and attachment to their ethnic group and shared racial values,

attitudes, and behaviors—were *less* likely to have a mental health problem over the course of their lifetimes.[10] Nonetheless, we are constantly self-monitoring and engaging in impression management, which can be exhausting.

This hypervigilance around what we say and do makes it difficult to be fully present and productive and negatively affects job performance. We run the risk of accepting the assumption (which indeed bodes merit in some circumstances) that we cannot bring our authentic selves to the workplace and in turn expend precious resources trying to figure out how to adjust appropriately. We may feel like we have to defend our competence and prove to others (and perhaps even ourselves) that we have a right to be present, seen, and heard. In response, we protect ourselves by not participating in the things that are meaningful in our lives in an attempt to avoid people and places where racism is most likely to occur.

Racism is making us sick, not just mentally, but also physically. We feel the ongoing, cumulative effects of racism strongly in our bodies. Researchers have found that experiencing, witnessing, or even hearing about racism and discrimination can result in the development of anxiety, depression, and post-traumatic stress disorder (PTSD).[11] Frequent experiences with racism and discrimination are associated with inflammation, which contributes to chronic illnesses such as asthma, arthritis, allergies, and cardiovascular disease. Dr. Sierra Carter and colleagues followed more than eight hundred Black families for almost twenty-five years and found that those who experienced higher levels of racial discrimination as teenagers were more depressed in their twenties and were aging at an accelerated rate on a cellular level.[12]

Even vicarious exposure to racism, such as media coverage of Black women being treated inhumanely and killed, can significantly impact stress and contribute to negative health outcomes. In the spring of 2020, we watched news cycles repeatedly cover the horrific story of twenty-six-year-old emergency room technician Breonna Taylor, who was shot and killed while sleeping in her own home during a botched police raid. Even after Taylor was recklessly shot, she did not receive any medical attention for more than twenty minutes. The police who killed her were not held accountable for her death but rather for "wanton endangerment" of the neighbors.

Just a few months after the death of Taylor, the story came to light of twelve male police officers who wrongfully entered the home of Anjanette Young with guns drawn and handcuffed her for more than forty minutes while she was naked. Young, a social worker, had just arrived home from work and was getting undressed for bed when the police barged into her home. A video taken from the officers' body cams shows Young naked, with her hands up, terrified and confused, telling the police more than forty times that they had the wrong home. During the dehumanizing event, the officers showed Young no respect or care for her human dignity.

These are only two examples of the ways that racism contributes to Black women being treated with suspicion, as a threat, and undeserving of decency or protection. When we watch such stories play out time and time again in the media, we are left intensely traumatized, and it is difficult to control worrying about our own safety and well-being as well as that of our loved ones. Many of us are walking around nervous and afraid all of the time.

Race-related stress and anxiety are further brought on by the realization that despite hard work, determination, and perseverance, we cannot control our own environmental contexts in order to guarantee fair and equitable treatment. We cannot control whether or not our talents, abilities, and character are seen or valued. The thought that despite jumping through all of the hoops we can still end up in unjust situations can leave us feeling powerless.

Through repeated encounters with racism and discrimination, we may consciously or unconsciously begin to accept negative and critical beliefs about our self-worth and feel hopeless about the likelihood of our circumstances improving. In turn, we have lower self-esteem, reduced belief in our ability to accomplish things, and lower life satisfaction. In order to stop this cycle, we must stop basing our sense of self-worth on success in spaces that do not support us, but rather be affirmed in the communities where we are fully accepted and valued. Identify these spaces and lean into them.

I have a friend, Nicole, who despite all of the challenges that life has thrown at her has been able to overcome and succeed professionally—like strong Black women do but not without considerable stress.

I first met Nicole when I was home for Christmas break of my freshman year in college. Her five-foot frame traipsed through the front door of our mutual friend's home atop four-inch pointy-toe stilettos. She took off her coat, unveiling an off-the-shoulder gray sequined cashmere sweater, tossed her freshly blown-out bouncy blonde hair, and took command of the room. With an open-mouthed laugh, she exuded a confidence that would later support her success as she climbed her way to the top of the corporate ladder.

After graduating from college with a bachelor of science degree in industrial engineering, Nicole went to work at a pharmaceutical company, where she had interned for three years. She had a job that she loved, with generous compensation and lots of perks. She was even on the fast track to becoming a manager. During the week she would fly first class across the country to her company's distribution centers to develop strategies to improve their operational excellence and efficiency. Her ambition earned her a personal relationship with the CEO, whom she had told during her internship that one day she would have his job.

On the weekends, Nicole scooped up her girlfriends in her cherry red Infiniti Q45 and used her art of seduction to get us into nightclubs without standing in line or paying cover charges. She drew men in and entertained them playfully. She was the boss in all situations. When she walked up, others stood to the side. Brazen fearlessness emanated from her. Living the life that she had always dreamed of, everyone, including me, admired her for her strength and ambition.

But along with her success came tremendous pressure and responsibility—family responsibilities, for instance. Nicole's mother struggled with mental illness and substance abuse, and as Nicole grew older and more independent, she frequently provided her with financial and emotional support. She was also the oldest of dozens of cousins and one of the first to go to college. Her success made everyone in her family look up to and turn to her in their times of need. When one cousin needed a loan to go to college, it was Nicole who cosigned. When another cousin needed a job after college, Nicole found her one at her company. And when yet another cousin found herself in a relationship with a violent man, Nicole stepped in to rescue her.

Nicole wanted to support her family, but she felt spread thin and overburdened. Her work travel schedule was grueling. She was taking care of everyone else and didn't have the time or energy to take care of herself. The multiple personal and professional demands that she faced impeded her self-care. When she was on the road, she ate out more and exercised and slept less.

When I asked Nicole what caused her stress, she said: "The

feeling that there are so many different dimensions that I need to be good at in order to be successful in my career and provide for my family. I feel the need to be a good mother, wife, career woman, and community advocate. I often worry that I'm not a great friend, connected enough to my extended family, or giving enough of my-self outside of my family. I see other women on social media and ask myself: Why am I not involved in more community activities? Why aren't my husband and I having exciting international travel adventures? Why am I not saving the world? The pressure to do it all causes me a lot of stress. It seems like I'm never doing enough."

We Black women often receive this message—that in some way, shape, or form, in big and in small ways, we aren't *doing* enough or we *aren't* enough. The media tell us that our kinky hair and curvy bodies aren't beautiful enough. Men on the street who tell us to "smile" and ask us, "What you mad about?" tell us that we aren't cheery and approachable enough. Our colleague who talks over us or repeats what we've already said tells us that our voices don't mat-ter and our ideas aren't valid enough. When year after year our co-workers call us by the name of the other Black woman in the office, our individuality is robbed. When we're continually passed over for promotions and raises, we're told that we don't work hard enough and we aren't smart enough. When we're put down, lied to, cheated on, taken from by our men and family, we're told we aren't worthy enough of love. In response to all of this, we try to work harder and do more, but what we really need is to reject the pressure to grind harder to prove our worth, stop looking for validation and reassur-ance from other people, and instead know unequivocally that *we are enough*, just as we are.

Nicole admits that the pressure she feels is self-imposed. She is driven to provide her three children with the home life and all of the educational, extracurricular, and cultural opportunities that she didn't have as the daughter of a teenage mother living in rural America. As a successful first-generation college graduate who escaped poverty, she *has* to win because her parents do not have the resources to catch her if she falls.

Strong, successful Black women like Nicole are holding up our communities, workplaces, and families, and they are doing it so well they make it look easy. But it's definitely not easy. As a community, we tend to ignore the stress that can come with success like Nicole's, and in turn, we miss seeing our sisters fully. We don't acknowledge the pressure associated with being the only Black woman out of one hundred people in leadership in a company with more than two hundred thousand employees. We underappreciate the weight of responsibility that comes with being the one person to whom family members turn when they need something. And when we don't see these things, we continue to ask for more and more from such women until they are depleted.

When a woman like Nicole is experiencing chronic stress, she feels wound up all of the time and unable to rebound and return to her baseline state of calm when a stressor has been alleviated. She is always in "fight or flight" mode—keyed up, on edge, and ready to respond to the next perceived threat or attack. In this activated state, she may experience shallow breathing, shaky hands, increased heart rate, or slowed digestion. These physical symptoms, which are triggered by an increase in the stress hormone cortisol in the body, negatively affect mental and physical health.

Chronic stress also increases the risk of sleep problems. When you're stressed, you might find yourself lying awake in bed, tossing and turning, with your mind going through your to-do list or racing with worries. Sleep is closely tied to mood; people with difficulty sleeping are more irritable, and have problems with attention and concentration, which can make it hard to be productive during the day. The National Institutes of Health recommends that adults get at least seven to eight hours of sleep every night to be well-rested.[13]

Stress is also associated with high blood pressure, stroke, heart attack, diabetes, adverse birth outcomes such as miscarriage and preterm birth, and a weakened immune system. More than 40 percent of Black women have high blood pressure, a major risk factor for cardiovascular disease. A study of more than ten thousand postmenopausal Black women found that those who experienced significantly stressful life events such as the death of a spouse, divorce, abuse, job loss, or major financial problems were more likely to have a cardiovascular event such as chest pain, stroke, heart disease, or congestive heart failure.[14] Not surprisingly, the life expectancy of Black women is three years shorter than that of white women (seventy-eight versus eighty-one).[15]

Stress and anxiety are closely linked and share many of the same symptoms—excessive worry or nervousness, irritability, difficulty with focus and concentration, sleeplessness, fatigue, increased heart rate, shallow breathing, upset stomach, and muscle tightness or tension. While stress is a response to a threat and usually triggered by a specific external event (such as arguing with your spouse or having a deadline at work), anxiety is a reaction to poorly managed stress.

Anxiety is characterized by excessive, difficult-to-control fear or worry about everyday situations (finances, family, safety) that persists for weeks, months, or even years; doesn't go away after the trigger has passed; and interferes with day-to-day functioning. Anxiety disorders are the most common mental health condition in the United States, affecting forty million adults (19 percent of the population), and women are twice as likely as men to have an anxiety disorder.[16] Research has shown that women who strongly identify with the strong Black woman prototype are more likely to experience anxiety, probably because of the higher rates of trauma in their lives.[17]

The typical way that a strong Black woman copes with stress is by distancing herself from uncomfortable emotions, such as denying a problem exists, pretending that things are normal, or hoping that a problem will go away on its own. We see these coping skills as "being strong" and "pushing through." Other behaviors can include escapism or avoidance acts, such as shopping, eating and sleeping too much, cleaning excessively, being a workaholic, obsessively focusing on doing for others, procrastinating, always being late, abusing alcohol, and taking recreational drugs like marijuana or abusing prescription medication like sleeping aids and painkillers. Take a moment and ask yourself if you do any of these things when you're feeling stressed.

Black women are often running on *autopilot*—going through the motions of carrying out daily responsibilities and obligations without paying attention. While on autopilot, we also can engage in unhealthy behaviors that contribute to poor health, simply as a matter of habit. These unhealthy behaviors direct attention away from the stress, which unfortunately gives problems opportunities to worsen and develop into even bigger problems such as anxiety and depression. When we do not notice when the mind and body are letting us know that we are stressed, we do not have the wherewithal to implement the necessary behaviors to take care of ourselves. How often in your typical day do you simply stop and check in with your mind and body?

Before she had the insight or ability to actively confront the sources of stress in her life, Nicole used food and alcohol to cope with stress. In the evenings she had an extra bowl of ice cream or a second or third glass of wine to "wind down," to relieve the tension in her mind and body, and to help her fall asleep. However, alcohol intake before bed can actually disrupt the sleep-wake cycle. Although many Black women abstain from alcohol (45–60 percent) or are infrequent drinkers (34–36 percent), stress increases the risk for more heavy drinking.[18] Rates of drinking tend to be higher among high-earning professionals. In times of stress, a person who typically has only one to two drinks socially on the weekends might slowly creep up to two to three drinks each night. The National Institute on Alcohol Abuse and Alcoholism recommends that women have no more than one drink per day.[19]

Overeating comfort foods that are high in calories, fat, and carbohydrates or snacks with high sugar and salt content is also an unhealthy way to manage stress. When we're stressed, we eat without paying much attention to what we are putting in our mouths, or whether we are even hungry. Black women may use food as a way to regulate their traumatic stress through distraction, avoidance, and escape of reminders of the trauma.[20] Instead of thinking about money problems, work stress, and family drama, we turn to food, which offers a temporary feel-good. We don't hold back on the fried chicken, BBQ ribs, macaroni and cheese, and pound cake because they taste so good in the moment and we don't want someone telling us yet another thing that we can't do or can't have. We want to treat ourselves. Food is one of the few pleasures that can feel within a Black woman's reach. It's another way to fill the void. As a result, many stressed Black women have excess weight: 81 percent of Black women are overweight or obese.[21] The stress hormone cortisol is not only associated with excessive belly fat, but also slows down fat metabolism and makes it more difficult to lose weight.

In a seminal 2010 study published by Dr. James Jackson and colleagues in the *American Journal of Public Health*, they found that Black adults who were stressed were more likely to engage in unhealthy behaviors such as smoking and alcohol use and to be obese.[22] The relationship between stress and depression was stronger for those who engaged in *none* of the unhealthy behaviors than it was for those who had engaged in the unhealthy behaviors. In other words, Black people who are stressed are *less* likely to be depressed because they cope with their stress via unhealthy behaviors, but unfortunately, this puts them at greater risk for chronic health conditions. The American Psychological Association's *Stress in America* survey revealed that 33 percent of Americans never discuss ways to manage stress with their healthcare providers.[23]

The *weathering hypothesis*, proposed by Dr. Arline Geronimus at the University of Michigan, states that Black people experience premature health declines as a result of the combined burden of repeated exposure to social and economic adversity such as racism, trauma, and poverty.[24] In a research study in which she measured health deterioration, or weathering, using ten biomarkers related to stress (such as blood pressure, cholesterol and triglyceride levels, and body mass index), she found that Black women had the greatest probability of having a high score when compared with Black men, white men, and white women; the gap in scores became especially pronounced after age thirty. By age forty-five, 50 percent of Black women had a score indicating a high degree of wear and tear on the physical body, and by age sixty-four, 80 percent of Black women had a high score.

Although the likelihood of having a high weathering score was greater for those who were poor, high scores among Black people were not fully accounted for by the higher proportion of Blacks who were poor. Non-poor Black women were at least twice as likely to have high scores as non-poor white women, which likely is due in part to their experiences with racial and gender discrimination. In their roles in the workforce, and in ensuring the social and economic survival of Black families, Black women face exposure to stressors that require a high level of coping, resulting in wear and tear on the physical body and detrimental health effects.

When Nicole tried to incorporate activities to help alleviate her stress, like hanging out with friends, going to the gym, reading, or planning downtime, she felt even more stressed because it took away time from other things that she felt were more important—things that she felt she *should* be doing. She felt stuck in a losing game of trying to figure out what she was going to sacrifice in order to give a little bit more to something else. It never seemed like she was making the right choice. Usually, she sacrificed herself.

Sometimes the mere act of turning your attention toward that which is stressful, is stressful. For Black people to name that racism at their jobs is their primary stressor because they are not valued by their employers, are not paid enough, or feel isolated and unsupported is stressful because the very thought of beginning to look for other work is overwhelming, and even if they did find another job, they have little hope that the circumstances would be any different. In the moment, it feels better to slam their eyes shut, put their heads down, and pretend that everything is "fine."

Naming our stress, and recognizing the impact that it has on us, is the first step to changing the things that are within our control in service of our mental and physical health and well-being. We often have more options available to us than we might think. In some cases, we may not be able to change a situation, but we can change how we *respond* to it. Listen closely to what your emotions are telling you about what's working and not working in your life.

When we don't pay attention to the stress in our lives, it can take over and ultimately control us. By not managing our stress, we give up our power. But taking proactive steps to do something allows us to feel in control of circumstances and reduces the stress.

Being *problem-focused* when managing general stress requires transitioning from avoidance and denial to actively confronting the source of stress. People who are problem-focused recognize, for instance, that they feel angry, frustrated, and overwhelmed when their work assignments pile up on their desk and creep into their home life, causing them to feel guilty about whether or not they are being a good parent. Such people take a few minutes to pause and calm down before they react with frustration. Then they have the clarity of mind to assess the situation, communicate their needs, prioritize the tasks, and ask for the support that they need.

A problem-focused strategy includes the following:

1. **Develop skills to self-regulate emotion**—learn how to calm your mind and body in the moment. Don't act out of impulse, but with intention (which doesn't mean ignoring or denying negative emotions).

2. **Use assertive communication**—use your words. Explicitly state how you feel using an "I" statement and directly ask for what you need.

3. **Practice good time management by prioritizing tasks and setting boundaries**—contrary to popular belief, we are not superwomen and we can't (nor should we) do it all. And even when we try to, something is going to pay the price by not getting done as

well. Pick and choose where you are going to allocate
your time. Start handing out *No*'s—a lot of them.

A problem-focused strategy means looking at stress with a
magnifying glass and confronting high-priority items head-on. It
means identifying that despite your ambitious career goals, it is
a priority to slow down so that you can take care of yourself and
spend time with the people you love. It means making a plan to address your financial troubles and get out of debt rather than ignoring unpaid bills. It means making the doctor's appointment that
you have put off for months. It means giving yourself permission
to say *No* to chairing your sorority service day for the third year
straight. Rather than looking at the extended list of things on your
plate, it means focusing on the first two to three things that feel
manageable at the time.

Of course, all the stress in Black women's lives can be intensified by systemic racism in the United States. Unfortunately, racism
will likely be a source of stress that continues to impact the lives
of Black women at work, financially, and in our communities for
decades to come. We must develop and maintain tools for coping
with racism, such as:

- Maintain a strong sense of self and racial pride
- Deeply embed ourselves in support systems that affirm
  our value and worth
- Acknowledge the stress that racism triggers, the truth of
  our experiences, and be compassionate with ourselves
- Resist internalizing any fault for the racist acts of others
- Limit avoidable cues and triggers (such as the news and
  social media)

- Seek pleasure, rest, and relaxation (don't let anyone steal our joy!)
- Allow ourselves safe space to process, but not ruminate on, events
- Manage the emotional labor that we put out (such as racism-splaining)
- Make choices based on what is valuable and meaningful to us

When you start looking at your stress closely, you might be tempted to start beating yourself up or putting yourself down. Notice such thoughts when they show up, and let them go. Be kind to yourself. Starting today, hold space for uncomfortable emotions without judgment or letting them consume you. When you intentionally confront that which has brought you suffering, you have the power to reshape the meaning of that experience rather than letting it define you. By attending to difficult emotions with compassion and placing them in their proper context, you diminish the control that they have on your life.

THREE

Intergenerational Trauma

When a child is born, I'm sure you've heard someone say, *She's been here before.* It's a phrase our elders may use to describe a child's demeanor or a look in their eyes that suggests they are somehow already familiar with the struggles life will present. We've also heard, whether in criticism or praise, *She's just like her mother* or *just like her father.* Intentionally or not, we use these descriptions to claim our connection and influence on those around us.

Multiple factors over the course of childhood through adulthood work together to shape and continuously reshape who we will ultimately become—our strengths and vulnerabilities. The biopsychosocial model of health and illness states that interactions between biological (genes), psychological (emotions, personality), and social (family relationships, neighborhood environment) factors affect the cause, manifestation, and outcome of mental and physical wellness or illness.

Our genetic makeup is determined by that of our parents. Mental health conditions such as PTSD, anxiety, and depression can be passed on through one's genes—they can be inherited. For example, a child who has a mother with PTSD has a 30 percent increased risk of having symptoms of traumatic stress.[1] Similarly, the heritability of depression is estimated at 50 percent and that for anxiety ranges from 30 to 67 percent.[2]

As we go through life, our biology interacts with our individual psychological and social-cultural factors to collectively contribute to mental health. For example, a person born to a mother with a history of trauma, with a timid personality, whose father dies unexpectedly to gun violence, and has limited family support is more likely to be anxious as an adult. On the other hand, a person born to a mentally well mother who has not experienced significant trauma and who has an adaptable and agreeable personality is more likely to recover from traumatic events they may confront.

Traumatic experiences among Black women are intergenerational and can date back to slavery. While enslaved, Black women's bodies were exploited for labor in the fields, domestic work at home, breeding more "property," and sexual assault by their white male masters. Slave owners exerted their power, control, and domination—the tools commonly used by sexual abusers—to victimize Black women. The historical legacy of enslavement is now a part of a collective trauma and cultural experience of mass suffering among Black women.

Since enslavement, the methods of oppression have been internalized and replicated within our own communities. The biological, emotional, and behavioral aftereffects of historical trauma continue to be passed down, including continuing cycles of abuse, normalization of violence, and the code of silence about abuse. As women confront traumas, they often repeat the unhealthy methods of coping that have been modeled to them, and in turn they endure the same harmful consequences.

Joy DeGruy has posited in her 2005 book, *Post-Traumatic Slave*

Syndrome, that Black people experience this syndrome as adaptive survival behaviors due to generations of oppression of enslaved people and their descendants. She suggests that patterns of behavior reflective of post-traumatic slave syndrome include poor self-esteem, feelings of hopelessness, depression, suspiciousness of negative motivation of others, propensity for anger and violence, and internalized racism. These maladaptive thoughts and behaviors originated as survival strategies in the context of slavery, followed by systemic and structural racism and oppression, and have continued to be passed down through generations long after they have lost their contextual value.

The early field of *epigenetics*—the study of changes in genes that are not caused by changes in the DNA sequence—suggests that the effects of trauma may be inherited; that is, trauma leaves a mark on the genes that is passed to future generations and has the potential to subsequently affect mental and physical health. For example, generations later, the descendants of enslaved Black women might experience more anxiety, depression, and heart disease because of changes that occurred in their ancestors' genes and were passed through the generations, even if they didn't directly experience a trauma themselves.

As I look at my own matrilineal line, I see a clear pattern of intergenerational trauma and consequential trauma-related behaviors. My great-grandmother, Lilly Belle, was born of a relationship between her mother, a Black tenant farmer, and a white landowner in the Deep South in the late 1800s. Her husband and the father of her three oldest children died young in his twenties. The father of her fourth child (my grandmother) and her fifth and sixth children lived down the road, but he preferred to acknowledge only his legitimate wife and children. She was on her own with six children to raise. The trauma that my great-grandmother experienced increased my grandmother's vulnerability to traumatic stress, anxiety, and depression long before she ever confronted trauma herself.

But in time, my grandmother did experience trauma. Her move to Chicago was precipitated by her divorce from her physically and verbally abusive alcoholic husband. He was a bricklayer and a bootlegger who sold shots of liquor to his neighbors out of his bedroom window. Once, my grandfather dragged my grandmother out of a car and wrestled her onto the ground, trying to take the car keys. She suffered two stillbirths before my mother was born. The day that my mother was born, my grandfather was nowhere to be found. To compound the abuse, this Korean War veteran was having an affair with a woman that he and my grandmother went to high school with who lived across the alley.

After the divorce, my grandmother never received any child support, and my grandfather rarely visited his daughter—my mother. My grandmother accepted the situation for what it was because she *didn't* need *him anyway*. She stuffed her feelings down and pretended that he no longer existed.

By the time Grandma arrived in Chicago, the residue of her trauma was beginning to show. She and my mom slept side by side in twin beds until my mother was nineteen years old. Physically, they were within arm's reach, but emotionally, there was a gulf of presumptive answers to unasked questions between them. Grandma emanated a bitter coolness, and she expressed her feelings through sharp words with the dull ache of chronic fatigue that must come from constantly being in survival mode and punctuated them with the irritation of being asked to give more than she desired.

My grandmother accumulated traumas, but she never owned them. Even though she tried to protect herself against being victimized, the threat of danger was perpetual. One routine evening, Grandma left work and got into her blue Cadillac when a twenty-something thug approached the car and asked her for directions. In an uncharacteristic moment, caught off-guard, she rolled down the window just enough for him to reach into the car and snatch her purse. The man ran off with the body of the bag, but she clung to the straps, which ripped off. Here was someone trying to take something from her, again. Instinctively she fought back, unwilling to concede defeat.

"Niggas took my purse," she told my mother and me with an anger that dominated her fear. She saved the tattered purse straps as a reminder against future attack. Next time, she would be ready.

Fifty percent of women in the United States have experienced at least one traumatic—shocking, scary, or dangerous—event at some point in their lives.[3] In my own research I have found that over 80 percent of Black women report experiencing at least one traumatic event. Black women experience the highest number of cumulative traumatic events in their lifetimes; physical and sexual assault are the most common.[4] *Traumatic stress* is the emotional residue that is left after exposure to a traumatic event. Fear during and shortly after a traumatic event is a natural coping response that is crucial for survival and protection against future harm. Most people recover from the fear associated with an acute trauma. However, some have lingering symptoms and go on to develop PTSD. Symptoms of PTSD include:

- Reexperiencing the trauma, such as through flashbacks or nightmares
- Avoiding people, places, or things that remind one of the trauma

- Having negative beliefs about oneself, such as shame, blame, or guilt
- Experiencing changes in mood such as depression, anxiety, irritability, or hypervigilance, that is, increased alertness and scanning the environment looking for potential threats

For people with PTSD, the fear response is more quickly triggered, less easily turned off, and generalized to situations that are only vaguely similar to the original trauma. Often, they experience intense fear even in nonthreatening situations. People who have been exposed to multiple traumas, like my grandmother—who experienced domestic violence, pregnancy loss, poverty, racial and gender discrimination, and robbery—are even more vulnerable to a poorly regulated fear response. They go to laborious and inconvenient lengths to take control of their environment in order to avoid being harmed again. Being in control makes a person who has experienced trauma feel more safe.

For example, a woman who has been assaulted might be reluctant to go to public places like the grocery store alone in the daytime. In order to have as much predictability as possible, she prefers to always take the exact same streets. If the road is blocked and she is forced to take a different route, the divergence from plans designed to keep her safe causes anxiety and a sense of being overwhelmed. If she spots someone from a distance who resembles a man who assaulted her, perhaps they are both short and bald, she panics. If and when a threat does occur, it confirms that the world is dangerous. It also justifies the excessive, restricting safety behaviors that she has put into place.

This type of behavior may make people feel more safe, but it controls their lives and robs them of their freedom. Avoiding places that are only loosely associated with the trauma maintains the belief that these places are dangerous. On the other hand, confronting these places with care provides the opportunity to have a different experience, which in turn dispels the fear.

When people begin to understand that the stifling fear connected to the thought that bad things are destined to happen is connected to past trauma, and the likelihood of the feared event actually occurring in the future is low, they can stop exchanging joy in the present for anticipatory fear. Ask yourself, on a scale of zero to one hundred, how likely is it that the thing that you intensely fear will actually happen?

Twenty percent of people who experience a trauma develop PTSD, and up to 70 percent experience significant symptoms that don't, however, meet the threshold for a PTSD diagnosis.[5] Black people are more likely than white people to develop PTSD. People who experience trauma earlier in life, who experience an intense, long-lasting trauma, or who have other mental health issues such as depression or anxiety are at greater risk for developing PTSD.

Black women who have experienced a trauma, and strongly internalize the strong Black woman mandate, may deny and push away the difficult emotions that come with the trauma and in turn have a *harder* time coping with their feelings. Like the typical strong Black woman, my grandmother was always in control. She didn't trust many people or let anyone get too close. She didn't show weakness or vulnerability by displaying warmth or affection. However, after the mugging, aside from work and church, she rarely drove anywhere alone.

Grandma distanced herself from reminders of her past and

wanted to be seen only for the life that she single-handedly created—after all, she graduated from college, found stable employment, purchased her own home, and achieved financial independence. But traumatic stress probably played a role in the way that she functioned in the world. I imagine that she might have struggled to reconcile persistent feelings of self-doubt that resulted from being in an abusive relationship with belief in her intrinsic worthiness validated by her achievements. Rather than embrace her traumatic past within a larger story of survival and success, she might have felt shame and judgment that prevented her from holding space for all parts of herself with compassion. The hurt from trauma hardened her, and the anger grew on top to form the tough exterior that protected her from the dangerous outside world. I'm sure you know women like this in your own family. You can feel their love and warmth trying to burst through a barrier that can be felt, but not seen.

Grandma moved through life without much reflection on all that she had been through—and all that she had accomplished. She kept moving forward, on autopilot. However, this armor likely prevented her from feeling the healing of self-compassion and the wholeness of being woven into loving, nurturing relationships. It prevented her from thoroughly experiencing the opportunities for joy that she had worked so hard to create. She never gave a window into the thoughts and feelings that she tightly contained; rather, she combated even the suggestion of struggle.

Like my grandmother, my mother also inherited a genetic vulnerability to traumatic stress and saw trauma-related anxiety modeled to her in her environment at home. Parents who have experienced trauma often have excessive feelings of fear and worry that an unnamed catastrophic event is going to happen, so they try to exert control over their children in an attempt to keep them safe from harm. This behavior is intended to protect children, but instead, the adults model anxiety and the children internalize the fears and worries of their parents as their own. The fears of the parents become the fears of the children. My mother took on my grandmother's fear and message: the world is a dangerous place and people are bound to disappoint you, so don't expect too much, and prepare to be let down.

The fears that are given to us weigh us down, slow us down, and prevent us from exploring and embracing life fully. We can become so preoccupied with fear telling us all of the bad things that *might* happen that we lose sight of the possibilities in the world that could be available to us if we relinquished that fear. We don't move too far out of our comfort, or "safety," zone: we don't take that trip we've been wanting to take; we don't apply for that exciting new opportunity; we don't make ourselves vulnerable in relationships. We let our fear outweigh our fantasy.

When we act from a space of trauma—by avoiding, denying, or numbing pain or by being "strong"—we are unknowingly repeating harmful behaviors. The unaddressed fear, anger, and self-deprecation embedded within trauma persist and are passed on.

We Black women are often nervous, on edge, and afraid that someone is out to hurt us because history has taught us that that is bound to happen. This fear makes us suspicious of others and makes it hard for us to trust, sometimes even with our own family.

Modulating the tension between letting go of excessive fear and worry, while simultaneously being aware of the disproportionate dangers that Black women and their children face, can feel like a game of Russian roulette. At times, it may seem better to have the anticipatory anxiety "just in case," regardless of how harmful it may be to the self, if it ultimately means keeping you and your family safe. But being afraid is uncomfortable and restricting. What would it feel like to put down the fear and set yourself free?

Within trauma lies anger. Anger is a natural survival instinct in the face of trauma. It can also be a common response to situations that are unfair (which are common experiences for many Black women) and in which you have been victimized (unfortunately, also common). Among Black women, anger is a trauma response to the rejection, abandonment, childhood sexual abuse, domestic violence, police brutality, poverty, and everyday racism we continually endure. We can feel angry because we believe that life has dealt us an unfair hand, nothing ever seems to come easy, and we realize how hard it is to create the life that we imagined when we were young.

This anger can reveal itself as aggressiveness, hostility, and coldness. While it may seem that we snap at the littlest things, it's not the little things, but rather the accumulation of everything that we have been through. Our anger is a defense mechanism; it is protective.

Anger can show up in parent-child relationships through harsh words (such as put-downs), behavior (such as spankings), or extreme punishments. In some cases the behavior might escalate to verbal or physical abuse. Children on the receiving end of the anger may feel rejected and may blame themselves for it, as my mother did. They may also start to model this anger and exhibit aggressive and delinquent behaviors.

Anger can be constructive because it can help people to cope with traumatic stress by giving them the energy to keep going; it shifts their attention, thoughts, and actions toward survival. On the other hand, it can be destructive by leading to substance abuse, aggressiveness toward others (anger turned outward), or self-harm (anger turned inward). Research has shown that anger is related to high blood pressure, stroke, heart attack, a weakened immune system, and even early death.[6]

Intergenerational trauma seeps into how we see ourselves. When we're repeatedly victimized, we can start to believe that something is wrong with us and somehow we deserve the hand that we have been dealt. We feel helpless and stuck, and it seems like there's no escape. It erodes our soul and self-esteem.

Rather than directly confront our trauma and its repercussions, we tend to hold it fiercely in secret, as a way of protecting ourselves from negative judgment and rejection by others. Research has shown that secrecy can lead people to be preoccupied with thoughts about the trauma and hypervigilant with regard to keeping the secret.[7] Not only are we working to keep other people from discovering the secret, but we are living with it and ruminating on it all of the time. This mental act can subsequently exacerbate depression, anxiety, and demoralization. By staying silent, we continue to be weighed down by these traumatic experiences.

It is possible to move through the hurt of trauma. The psychological theory of post-traumatic growth explains the transformative growth that can come after a trauma. As a result of having endured an experience that shakes us to our core and causes intense emotional distress, and the struggle to move past it, we can come to see ourselves in a new way and understand the world differently. We might see ourselves as stronger than we thought; we might take steps to strengthen meaningful relationships in our lives, deepen our spirituality, and have a new appreciation for life. Given the multifaceted trauma that Black women continue to face, post-traumatic growth offers the possibility that instead of being stuck in suffering, our struggle can lead to emotional evolution.

A first step in breaking the cycle of intergenerational trauma is to acknowledge the traumas that exist in our families, the hurt that has grown from them, and the damage that they have caused us. For some people, a part of addressing familial trauma might include confronting people who have caused you harm (perhaps unknowingly) and letting them know how their behavior made you feel. Know that your feelings are valid whether or not the other person acknowledges them. This should only be considered in situations where you feel physically and emotionally safe, otherwise you may risk being retraumatized. Separate the process of communicating your feelings from the outcome—the person may not be ready to accept their role in the trauma and in turn may not respond how you'd like. Then forgive them. Forgiveness allows you to free yourself from the anger that is eroding you and holding you back.

In order to learn and grow, we must invite our elders to engage us in open conversations about their experiences, rather than maintain the tradition of not questioning. When we recognize the unhealthy patterns of behavior that have been passed down to us and that we might pass down to our children, we can liberate ourselves from harmful routines and choose a different path forward. Dismantling the code of silence around abuse opens us up to be able to share stories to educate and protect the next generation of girls and free them from shame. When we speak out these stories, with our sisters who share them, we lighten the collective load.

FOUR

Loss of Innocence

Many Black women have endured physical and sexual abuse as children.[1] Well-known, successful women like Alice Walker, Maya Angelou, and Oprah Winfrey have shared the ways that their personal experiences with childhood sexual abuse impacted their self-esteem and romantic relationships, and how they were ultimately able to heal from the trauma and thrive.

Winfrey, who has repeatedly been named as one of the world's most powerful women, was born into poverty and had a teenage mother. When Winfrey was nine years old, she was raped by her cousin. She was also sexually abused by her uncle and a family friend. When she was fourteen, she prematurely gave birth to a baby boy who died shortly thereafter. When speaking about how she moved past her traumas, Winfrey said, "When we hold secrets it creates shame, and shame is a great barrier to success. When you carry the shame, you do not allow yourself to fulfill your greatest potential." Releasing the shame and telling their stories has helped so many Black women see that they are not alone. Although trauma may be a part of your story, it doesn't have to define it.

Childhood sexual abuse includes any contact between an adult and a child, or an older child and a younger child, for the purposes of sexual gratification for the older person. It can happen with anyone who has easy access to a child—older siblings, extended family members, teachers, coaches, a parent's partner, even a parent. The vast majority, 90 percent, of sexually abused children know their abuser; 60 percent are abused by someone the family trusts; and a third are abused by a family member.[2] Child sexual abuse ranges from child pornography, exposing oneself to a child, obscene phone calls, fondling, oral sex, or penetration. Incest is the most common form of child sexual abuse. To be clear: a child can never truly "consent" to any form of sexual activity; child sexual abuse takes advantage of children's vulnerability and robs them of their innocence.

Some perpetrators gain the trust of children by slowly grooming them over time, in an attempt to form a close relationship. They pay children special attention, fill their unmet needs (financial, attention, validation), isolate them from others, treat them as if they are older, gradually cross physical boundaries, and use secrecy, blame, and threats to maintain control.

Less than 38 percent of child victims disclose that they have been sexually abused, even if they are explicitly questioned.[3] For children who do not disclose their abuse, or do not have a nurturing support system, distorted thoughts about themselves and the accompanying negative emotions can become deeply embedded in their identity. A believing and supportive caretaker can be a strong determinant for a good prognosis following abuse.

The reluctance of children to disclose abuse usually stems from fear of the perpetrator, concern that they will not be believed, or the potential consequences of telling, which can leave children feeling trapped and helpless. Victims of child sexual abuse can be confused as to whether or not abuse actually occurred, particularly if there was no intercourse, an older child was involved rather than an adult, or they felt pleasure from the experience. People may also question whether they were actually abused if they cannot clearly remember details of what happened. This can occur if they *dissociate*, that is, "go away" in their heads or black out as a way of tolerating the painful feelings that otherwise feel too difficult to bear. Dissociation can also include flashbacks, nightmares, and emotional numbness.

It is not unusual for victims of child sexual abuse to deny that they were abused, that the abuse caused them any harm, or that they need help. They experience the contradictory feeling that something "wrong" happened even though they trust the authority of the abuser. When the abuse is perpetrated by someone whom victims look up to, it can be hard for them to see the perpetrator in a negative light, making it even more difficult for them to see the abuse as not their fault. Victims have difficulty externalizing the abuse and in turn internalize it and think negatively about themselves. Consequently, admitting abuse would come with feelings of shame, self-blame, and guilt since they believe that they must have caused it to happen.

Children in poorer households are three times as likely to be the victims of child sexual abuse. The risk of sexual abuse is tripled for children whose parents are not working.[4] Children who live with a single parent or a stepparent are also at an increased risk for child sexual abuse. Two-thirds of Black children live with a single mother. Single parenthood more than doubles the risk of the involvement of Child Protective Services and is the second largest predictor of child maltreatment, after income. Children who live with a single parent who has a live-in partner are twenty times more likely to be victims of childhood sexual abuse than children living with both biological parents. About one in ten Black mothers cohabitates with a partner. Children in families with an unstable family structure, or a lot of family conflict, including domestic violence, are also at greater risk for maltreatment. A parent's history of child abuse, mental illness, or substance abuse can further increase the likelihood of childhood abuse.[5]

The groundbreaking study "Girlhood Interrupted: The Erasure of Black Girls' Childhood" found that adults view Black girls in the age range of five to fourteen as less innocent and more adult-like than their white peers.[6] Black girls were also perceived to need less nurturing and protection; to know more about adult topics, including sex; and to be more independent. The follow-up study, "Listening to Black Women and Girls: Lived Experiences of Adultification Bias," found that negative stereotypes of Black women such as being angry and aggressive or hypersexualized are placed onto Black girls and in turn erase the distinction between childhood and adulthood.[7] These perceptions of Black girls likely play a role in their heightened vulnerability to childhood sexual abuse.

Gloria, Angel, and Heaven are three women I worked with in therapy who experienced childhood sexual abuse. Let's meet Gloria first. For at least the first year of therapy, Gloria sat across from me with her eyes resting down in her lap. She kept her long trench coat and hat on in the office, preventing any skin from showing aside from her face, neck, wrists, and hands. When she spoke, she covered her mouth. She was careful about what she said and periodically peeked up to search my face for signs of approval or rejection.

In the first session, Gloria disclosed that she had been raped by her father from the ages of seven to thirteen. Every time her mother prepared to leave home, she clung to her waist out of fear of what would happen when she was alone with her father. She wanted her mother to stay and protect her.

Gloria's mother worked as a missionary and spent her days saving souls. Then she came home to her own hell on earth. She knew Gloria's father was abusing Gloria but took no apparent steps to try to stop it.

Gloria was also molested by her cousin, a friend of the family, and later her mother's boyfriend. She didn't bother telling her mother about it because she didn't think that it would matter and feared that her mother would blame her for letting it happen and accuse her of being "fast."

When Gloria told me about the abuse, she had no emotion. Her words flowed seamlessly in a monotone voice. She described the details as if she were telling me a story about someone else. These events certainly had happened, but she seemed to have inoculated herself from the distant memory and the suffering within.

As a way of coping with the abuse, Gloria overate to make herself less attractive. She reasoned that being fat would protect her from people getting too close. It worked, somewhat. She was bullied in school because of her weight and didn't have any friends. (Children who are abused are more likely to become obese in middle age.) Later, when Gloria was sixteen, a twenty-one-year-old man in the neighborhood started to notice her and spend time with her. "He was nice to me," she said. Desperate to escape the abuse at home, she moved in with her charming and attentive boyfriend, and when she was seventeen, they married.

Angel's story is much the same. She was sexually abused by multiple men from ages three to sixteen. Several factors in her life made her more vulnerable to abuse. She was born to teenage parents—her mother was fifteen and her father, eighteen. Her home environment was chaotic as her mother sold crack out of the home and cycled boyfriends in and out. Preoccupied by her own distress,

Angel's mother was unavailable to provide Angel with the attention or affection that she needed. However, Angel's grandmother stepped in and did the best that she could to help raise her. Angel never told her mother about the abuse.

The relationship between Angel's parents dissolved quickly, and her father married and started another family. When her father was deployed to military service in Germany, in the midst of Angel's abuse and neglect at home, her feelings of rejection and abandonment were solidified. She believed that her father loved her, but she was angry that she was not allowed to go away with him. She acted out by getting into fights, skipping school, stealing, and engaging in sexually promiscuous behavior. At age eighteen Angel moved in with her boyfriend, and she soon became pregnant.

Then there's Heaven, who was raped by her father's friend and molested by her grandfather. When I met Heaven, she was thirty-four years old and drenched in sorrow and despair. Heaven's short round frame sank into the couch, and she kept her dusty black puffy coat on with her arms tightly folded around her waist for the hour-long session. She was literally trying to hold herself together.

Heaven was also born to a teenage mother. She was passed around among the homes of her mother, grandmother, and aunt, but most often, she was left to roam the streets and care for herself. She, too, acted out by being promiscuous. And when she got pregnant at sixteen, she also moved in with her twenty-one-year-old boyfriend.

These stories might sound familiar to you because even though we don't often talk about childhood sexual abuse, it is all too common. Nonetheless, the overwhelming majority of Black women who have experienced child sexual abuse never receive support or counseling from a mental health provider. By keeping these experiences secret, even as adults, we are walking around with the baggage and leaving the wounds unhealed. But when we confront these experiences and share our stories, we give ourselves an opportunity to work through the pain.

Kim Foxx, the first Black woman to hold the office of State's Attorney for Cook County, Illinois, is a beautiful example of someone who has been able to move from trauma to triumph. Every year, more than 3.6 million referrals are made to Child Protective Services nationwide, and more than 700,000 children experience substantiated abuse.[8] In Cook County, the Office of the State's Attorney is responsible for taking legal action on cases of child abuse after they have been investigated and substantiated by the Department of Children and Family Services. Over the years, I've had the opportunity to get to know Foxx and develop a friendship through meetings at various community events. Her unabashed openness drew me to her.

Foxx experienced childhood sexual abuse first when she was six years old and molested by a teenage cousin. She was confused that someone who was a part of her family, whom she had affection for, was doing something that didn't feel right. A lot of sexual play went on between cousins back then, and she hadn't yet developed the capacity to know that what was happening to her was outside of the norm. Her childhood innocence was preyed upon and taken advantage of.

Foxx's mother discovered the abuse when she found semen in her daughter's panties while doing the laundry. She confronted her with a tone that was both accusing and protective—looking her in the eyes, gripping her shoulders and shaking her, and demanding, "Who hurt you?" She then stormed out of the house to go "fuck up" that cousin. She had not been able to protect her daughter in the moment, but she was on the way to find street justice.

When Foxx was seven, she met sexual violence again. Two boys raped her in an abandoned building near the Cabrini-Green housing projects in Chicago where she lived. Shortly thereafter, probably as a result of the abuse, she started masturbating to stimulate the sexual arousal that had been prematurely awakened in her, and she developed a heightened interest in boys.

During her freshman year in college, Foxx was violated for a third time when she went to a guy's dorm room late at night. He started getting handsy, and she felt uncomfortable, but she didn't want to offend him or hurt his feelings. Fear of rejection or punishment led her to put his needs before her own. She didn't want to have sex, but she asked herself, *If you didn't want this, why did you come here in the first place?* She didn't fight or scream. As a child she didn't have the capacity to consent, and as an adult she felt powerless to deny her consent. She felt ashamed and disappointed and blamed herself for letting it happen.

After Foxx had been assaulted three times, the feelings of worthlessness that too often accompany abuse settled into her identity. She started to believe that she had deserved it and thought, *This is who I really am.*

Foxx has been outspoken about her personal experience with multiple childhood traumas, none of which were ever reported, investigated, or prosecuted. In addition to child sexual abuse, she was exposed to domestic violence in her mother's relationship, and she grew up in public housing where she was surrounded by poverty and gun violence. She was raised by a single mother who suffered from untreated bipolar disorder. Yet she still had the protective support of her grandmother, a strong Black woman, who helped her mother raise her after her father had left the home. Foxx's grandmother taught her how to be strong and instilled in her confidence, dignity, and the sense that she was enough, despite her circumstances.

When Foxx talks about her trauma, she exemplifies the power within vulnerability that is uncovered when you let go of shame and courageously honor and accept all aspects of your personal journey without judgment. Her self-assuredness is deeply felt when she talks with confidence and apparent ease about how her life experiences have shaped her and make her uniquely qualified to do her job. She affirms her self-worth in being unapologetic about who she is and where she comes from.

Typical of many strong Black women, when Foxx walks into a room, she takes control of it. She holds her head high and looks people in the eye with love and understanding in a way that conveys *I see you*. She puts definitive periods behind her bold statements, leaving little room for anyone to contest that it is indeed possible to be redeemed from even the most devastating of circumstances.

Yet the remnants of her abuse lie in a corner space of her authority. Every blue moon, the darkness of being molested by her cousin returns to her, and she can see and smell an unidentifiable, glistening penis. It makes her want to gag. This reexperiencing is unpredictable and jarring. Sometimes it happens when she is trying to be intimate with her husband, and other times, when she is simply reading a book.

Foxx confronts reminders of her trauma daily through her work. Once, when she heard a young attorney ask, "What kind of mother lets their children watch them get beat up?," it felt like a personal attack on her own mother. When she was working on a case of a thirteen-year-old girl whose stepfather was touching her while having sex with the mother, she saw herself in the young girl who was visibly broken. When underage girls who claimed that the famed singer R. Kelly sexually abused them were not believed, the shame and embarrassment from the precarious night in that guy's college dorm room returned.

Foxx finds meaning and purpose in her life experiences through her work as State's Attorney. Not only is she at the helm of protecting and wielding justice for thousands who have been the victims of child abuse, sexual assault, and domestic violence, but she is a living example of surviving and thriving. She uses the empathy garnered through her trauma history to serve as an advocate for young girls who are wrestling with feelings of worthlessness and on the brink of giving up hope.

However, at times her work serves as a distraction from the harbored pain she inevitably feels. She holds the fact that her presence has value in the forefront of her mind and puts her personal suffering to the rear in order to be a vehicle of healing for others. This practice allows her to be strong and keep going. This is one of the many ways in which she is self-sacrificing.

In order to address the residual effects of her trauma, Foxx has started therapy. Her therapist encourages her to confront her trauma history, notice the ways that it shows up in her day-to-day life, and prioritize taking care of herself. She encourages Foxx to revisit the scared little girl who still lives deep inside and to answer the question, *What about* your *needs?*

Few stories highlight the way that vulnerable Black girls are preyed upon better than that of the once revered, now defamed singer R. Kelly.[9] After the evidence against him had mounted for decades, and in the light of the six-part documentary *Surviving R. Kelly* being aired, it was State's Attorney Kim Foxx who asked for anyone with sexual allegations against him to come forward.[10]

Kelly has been accused of abusing women and girls over the

past twenty years; the charges against him include child pornography, enticement of a minor to engage in sex, sexual exploitation of children, aggravated criminal sexual abuse, sex trafficking, and kidnapping. The accusations against him sit at the complex intersection of child sexual abuse and intimate partner violence and provide a chilling illustration of the tactics of control, manipulation, and intimidation employed by perpetrators of violence, and the potential long-lasting psychological implications for the victims.

In 1994, twenty-seven-year-old Kelly married the fifteen-year-old singer Aaliyah, who reportedly claimed she was eighteen. Although the relationship was questioned by the media and the general public, it was not readily perceived as predatory or objected to, and Kelly suffered no obvious consequences. Many people, including myself, sang right along to Aaliyah's "Age Ain't Nothing but a Number" and affirmed their own questionably appropriate relationships with older men. In the years following Kelly's marriage to Aaliyah, he was sued by several other women who accused him of having an inappropriate sexual relationship with them when they were underage. These cases were ultimately settled out of court with a monetary payment to the alleged victims, and Kelly's legendary status remained intact.

When I was in high school in Chicago in the 1990s, Kelly could regularly be found outside of his alma mater, Kenwood Academy, leaning against his white Mercedes Benz and wearing dark sunglasses. Crowds of naive and impressionable teenage girls swarmed around him, hopeful to catch a glimpse of the star, or if they were lucky, to be chosen. To be noticed by Kelly would validate their specialness, a reassurance that so many teenage girls seek. Kelly was known to lurk around places where young girls were easily accessible, like the South Side YMCA and Oak Park and River Forest High School.

The girls whom Kelly victimized shared common characteristics: they were young, impressionable, and showed signs of low self-esteem. Many of them were shy, came from troubled homes with strained finances, and dreamed of making it big as singers. To have a close and personal relationship with someone as revered as Kelly meant everything to them.

But Kelly manipulated them by using his age, status, and money and their interest in the music business to draw them close, make them feel special, and establish an unhealthy power dynamic. He used his power to control their behavior by dictating when they ate, when they bathed, and who they interacted with. They were isolated from friends and family and in turn completely dependent on him. After years of mind control, manipulation, and intimidation tactics, the girls and women lost sight of themselves and their own power. They believed that they couldn't leave.

Women who have experienced chronic abuse are vulnerable to entering a state of *learned helplessness*, in which they feel powerless and eventually give up on the possibility of escape. As a result of the abuse, their low self-esteem becomes cemented with the rationalization that if they had any worth and value, people wouldn't be treating them the way they are being treated. They can also be riddled with feelings of self-blame, guilt, and fear of being abused again. Women can be so overcome with intense anger and frustration that they harm themselves—excessively using drugs and alcohol, engaging in risky sex, mutilating their bodies, or even attempting suicide. On the other hand, women might cope by becoming numb, not feeling much of anything at all.

Although child sexual abuse among Black girls often goes unnoticed and untreated, the signs may be present, and it is important that parents are equipped with the information to recognize those signs. Children who have been sexually abused often have physical signs such as bruising or swelling of the genitals, sexually transmitted infections, or even broken bones. There may be bloodstains on sheets or undergarments. Additionally, such children are prone to myriad short- and long-term behavioral and psychological consequences. They may demonstrate a decline in academic performance and an increase in delinquency/conduct problems, such as aggressive behavior and fighting at school. Thoughts about the abuse can be distracting and lead to impaired attention, concentration, and difficulty in learning. Adolescent victimization, which Black girls are at greater risk for, reduces the odds of employment in adulthood by 51 percent.[11]

Abused children can also be clingy, not wanting to be left alone with certain people, or they may want to spend an unusual amount of time alone. They demonstrate inappropriate sexual knowledge or behavior, such as fondling, pelvic thrusting, and masturbation. Given child survivors' state of psychological distress, they are more likely to engage in risky sexual behaviors, such as unprotected sex with multiple sexual partners. As a result, they have higher rates of teen pregnancy. Forty-five percent of pregnant teens have had a past experience of childhood sexual abuse.[12]

Other signs of sexual abuse are behavioral changes, such as children shrinking away from physical contact; returning to regressive behaviors, such as bed wetting or thumb sucking; or becoming overly protective of other siblings. Their eating habits, sleeping patterns, or hygiene routines may also change—such as refusing to bathe or bathing excessively.

Survivors of child sexual abuse may struggle to reconcile feeling both defiled and special. They often feel ugly and dissatisfied with their bodies or appearance. As Gloria did, they may overeat, be obese, or have other eating disorders. They often have difficulty with trust in relationships, which affects their ability to be vulnerable and to engage in a healthy sexual relationship.

Sexually abused children are vulnerable to developing depression and anxiety and having suicidal thoughts. The abuse causes them to be excessively fearful and worried for a period of time that can last long after the abuse has ended. Low self-esteem that begins in childhood can persist into adulthood. Feelings of anger and resentment may be present for caregivers whom they believe abandoned them and did not protect them.

Black mothers, especially those who have experienced abuse themselves, may be so afraid of their daughters being victimized that they avoid talking about sex, or they may give threatening commands that instill fear: *Stay away from boys! Don't have sex! Keep your legs closed!* or *Don't you bring home no baby!* Girls might be passively taught that sex is bad but not be given information on what to do with their sexual urges or how to protect themselves if they choose to become sexually active or find themselves in a situation in which they are being sexually coerced or forced.

In an attempt to protect young girls' innocence, adults may use euphemistic words to talk about body parts—such as *pocketbook* instead of *vagina*. This can further confuse children. Research has shown that teaching children the proper names of their body parts and that some parts of their bodies are private and shouldn't be touched or looked at can help protect them against abuse.[13] It's also helpful to teach children that it is okay to say *No* when someone touches them in a way that makes them feel uncomfortable (even if it is a family member).

A first step in addressing Black girls' vulnerability to childhood sexual abuse is for parents to minimize opportunities for children to be abused by eliminating or reducing isolated, one-on-one social situations in favor of group situations where multiple adults supervise children. Parents should also pay close attention to their children and watch out for sudden changes in their moods or behaviors. If you are concerned that your child may have been abused, ask them about it directly. Do so in a calm and even tone. Assure them that they won't be blamed or punished. Listen to their response.

Create a space that is safe and comfortable to have open conversations with children about their bodies and sex. When appropriate, talk to them about sexuality and explain what sexual abuse is. Teach them how to establish and maintain physical and emotional boundaries and to tell a trusted adult if anyone violates those boundaries. Encourage them to come forward if something happens that they have been taught is not right or makes them uncomfortable—even if they have been told to keep it a secret.

If you notice signs of abuse, or have suspicions, act responsibly and take action. It is time to take action if a child has disclosed abuse, if you discovered abuse on your own, or if you suspect it. In cases of disclosure or discovery, report the abuse to local law enforcement or Child Protective Services. If you've discovered child pornography, report it to the police or to the CyberTipline of the National Center for Missing and Exploited Children at www.cyber tipline.org.

Additional resources include the National Sexual Violence Resource Center (nsvrc.org), the Rape, Abuse & Incest National Network (RAINN; rainn.org), and the National Child Traumatic Stress Network (NCTSN; nctsn.org).

INTIMACY

"Your silence will not protect you."

AUDRE LORDE

FIVE

Relationship Baggage

People often unconsciously search for a mate who has traits their parents had. Those familiar traits, both positive and negative, help the relationship feel comfortable and provide an opportunity for people to heal emotional and psychological damage they experienced in childhood. But by picking the same type of person, they also can be chronically reinjured.

My mother unconsciously fell into this pattern of trying to repair the wounds left by the negative traits of her father by picking partners who possessed similar traits. Without ever having a model for a healthy intimate relationship, she, like many of us, was lost in trying to get one. Her first boyfriend was Luther Wallace. Ten years older than my mother, he was the assistant manager at the local supermarket where she worked part time while she was in school part time. He was tall and heavy set and loomed over my petite and curvy mother. He wore his straight jet-black hair combed to the back. The bottom of his front tooth was jagged and especially noticeable when he would call anyone within spitting distance of his tongue "D.A.," for dumbass.

My mother was accustomed to his verbal lashings and had

grown a thick skin to deflect them. Luther customarily indulged in whisky, but according to her, he could hold his liquor "pretty good."

One summer weekend my mother told my grandmother, with whom she was still living, that she was going on vacation with Luther. When my mother returned, the locks on the house had been changed. My grandmother thought if her daughter was grown enough to go on vacation with her grown-man boyfriend, then she no longer needed to live under her mother's roof.

On her own for the first time, my mom rented a room where she stayed when she wasn't at Luther's place. Initially, he was a good presence in her life. He supported her financially while she was in school. Luther taught her to drive and let her borrow his car when she needed it. However, after a few years, she realized that there was something Luther couldn't give her—the family that she wanted. He had been married before and already had kids, and he didn't want to do either again. So, with little reservation, she ended the relationship.

By then, she was in her late twenties and thought, *Nobody wants to marry me.* Despite the general consensus by both men and women that she was "fine," she didn't see herself as particularly desirable. Then she met Ray Robinson. He was tall and smooth, and when he flashed his crooked smile, the gold that trimmed his front teeth sparkled.

But Ray was also older than my mother—twenty years this time—and divorced, with two children. He was more amenable to the idea of marriage than Luther had been, which was one of the more attractive things about him. Ray was fun, but her feelings for him were lukewarm at best. She was not easily lured into the promise of happy endings and was accustomed to disappointment, so she guarded her feelings closely and tempered her expectations.

After a year, and unbeknownst to my grandmother, Mom and Ray got married at the courthouse with modest enthusiasm and no ring, dress, or fanfare. The relationship had been strained even before it became legal, as Ray fancied the thrill of gambling—horses, cards, and dice. When he wasn't working, he was gambling away his money, and Mom was left with the sole responsibility of paying the bills. She was so outraged by his behavior that she repeatedly asked him to get out of their townhome. He arrogantly refused, telling her that he wasn't "payin' nothin'" and he wasn't "goin' nowhere."

After an unlucky night gambling, Ray came home late to my angry mother. They exchanged a series of back-and-forths about what he was and wasn't gonna do, and then he slapped her. Grandma and her man-friend Cliff came over to assess the situation and took my mother home with them. Grandma, who thought my mother would be better off with a boyfriend than a husband, gave her the money to get a lawyer and a divorce.

Mom didn't give too much thought to the commonalities in her relationships—handsome, charming, older, emotionally unavailable men, with limited capacity to give her the commitment and family that she wanted. Without any awareness of the pattern of the type of men to whom she was drawn, she continued in a cycle of repeating the same behaviors.

At a time when Mom was forlorn and vulnerable, she met my dad at the school where she was working. He was the principal, and Mom was a substitute teacher. Physically, he resembled the men who'd come before him—tall, with deep brown skin. He glided down the school hallways purposefully with a stern expression that commanded obedience. He was also thirteen years her senior, married, and had a child.

When my dad moved on to open a new school, he took my

mother with him and gave her a teaching job—her first. Initially, she wasn't interested in having a relationship with him. She was still grieving her recent divorce and had just about given up on finding love and having a family of her own. But he was persistent in his pursuit, despite being married. He took her to nice dinners, bought her designer purses and shoes, and gave her a Neiman Marcus credit card. He romanced her with flowers, cards, and poetry. He told her that he loved her—words that she'd rarely, if ever, heard from anyone.

Is this what love looks like? she wondered. She was ambivalent about the prospect. She admired his confidence and knowledge of the world. He had more to offer her than the men who'd come before, even if it wasn't everything that she sought. He attended to her in a way that no one else ever had and fed the loneliness and feeling of not being good enough that had been planted and sown since she was a little girl.

Although she had given up on getting married again, she still wanted to have a child. She told herself, *This is all that I need. This will make me happy.* But subconsciously, she may have felt, *This is all that I deserve.* Her own father hadn't shown her what a consistent presence and unconditional love look like in a relationship with a man, so why should she expect that from anyone else? Relatively speaking, her present situation was better than her previous relationships. So she put together a family, into which I was born, with what seemed like the best option at the time.

Dad would spend evenings with us, but after he left to go home to his wife and child, Mom's contentment would shift. The fulfilling part of the night was concluded, and the ordinary and habitual began. She futzed around the kitchen and living room, wiping off countertops, arranging and rearranging. She switched off the lights glowing through the crystal seashell chandelier that hung above the dining room table. Darkness covered her in the now deflated space. There was nothing more for her to do, and no one to talk to. Her eyes gazed out the window, and her thoughts ran aimlessly. Silence was loud and said things that she didn't want to hear. Later, alone in her bedroom, she flicked on the television to distract her attention and keep her company.

My mother's father had been physically distant and emotionally unavailable. He hadn't given her much attention or validation. He didn't model for her what healthy, reliable love from a man looks like. When she found herself in relationships that didn't meet her needs as an adult, she accepted them as the familiar norm. She didn't believe that she had the power to ask for, or expect, more.

Relationship problems are among the most common issues that cause women distress. Strained relationships with their fathers, or a string of unsuccessful intimate relationships, may leave them feeling flawed, damaged, and unlovable. They may wonder, *What's wrong with me? What am I doing wrong?* Even those who seem to be doing everything "right" in terms of trying to find a partner—doing the self-work, being open-minded, putting themselves out there— can feel shame and embarrassment if all that energy doesn't result in a fulfilling relationship. They internalize the "failure" as meaning that something is inherently wrong with them.

Many Black women have been conditioned with old wives' tales about what they need to do in order to get and keep a man. We're taught that we have to cook, clean, parent the children, cater to the man, and have enough energy left over to be on call in the bedroom. We have to look a certain way—so we go on crash diets or surgically alter our bodies in order to meet the beauty standard that we believe men expect. We have to act a certain way, too—submissive, accommodating, and not too demanding. In the process of trying to be with someone, we shrink our true selves in order to make room for someone else. Even in relationships, we are tricked into thinking that we have to do the bulk of the giving, rather than receiving.

This is what I'm supposed to do, we tell ourselves. *This is my duty as a girlfriend or wife.* And honestly, many of the elder women in our lives reinforce this message. As a result, we're stressed trying to be perfect, create the picture-perfect household, and avoid doing something that will make our man run off. Because if that happens, surely we'll be the one to blame.

On the other hand, single women can ache with loneliness and get lost in the fantasy of what their lives would be like if they had that idealized partner. *He's got to be six-foot-two, have a six-figure income, look good in a suit, but can also get under the hood of a car, love the Lord, give back to the community, and for sure be able to rock my world.* A woman can imagine all of the fun things that she and her partner will do together when they *finally* find each other—the date nights they'll have, the trips that they'll take, and even what their future children will look like. But while in dreamland, she passes by opportunities for happiness in the moment.

When this supposedly ideal person proves to be less than ideal, she is unwilling to flex her standards because that's how it's *supposed* to be. She becomes hopeless and drops down into despair with the realization that the dream she clings to isn't her reality. Then when another potential candidate doesn't work out, her self-esteem plummets more. Anxiety-driven worry floods in, and she starts to fear being alone and lonely the rest of her life.

Indeed, research has found that loneliness is associated with mental health conditions like anxiety, depression, cognitive decline, and physical conditions like high blood pressure and heart disease.[1] However, often when people feel lonely, they are unable to see and embrace the love that is actually present in their lives. Yes, I understand, friend and family love is not the same as intimate love. But when we discount the presence of love that does exist, we rob ourselves of its comfort.

Despite wanting the perfect relationship, time after time we can find ourselves choosing the wrong person. We fall into the trap of the charming ladies' man, flattered by the attention and convincing ourselves that we're the one he'll settle down with. In turn, we become frustrated as we try to adjust ourselves, or force him to change, in order for the relationship to work. We pick the guy who "looks good on paper," but we don't have the chemistry or emotional connection that we need. We pick the guy who's not bringing that much to the table, leaving us to pick up the slack, because being next to a warm body beats being alone. Then there's the pressure of the biological clock if we want to have children, which can lead us to make additional sacrifices and concessions in our selection of a mate.

We play mind games with ourselves, exaggerating the positives and minimizing the negatives in order to rationalize the dubious choices that we make. Having a man can be seen as a badge of honor, and when we don't have one, well, we've lost. All the while we are trying to meet the pressure filled expectations of what we believe our lives are supposed to look like.

When you are looking for a relationship, it is important to take the time to really get to know yourself, your strengths, your vulnerabilities, and behavioral patterns—and a therapist can help with this. This crucial first step, which often comes after a significant period of self-reflection while not in a relationship, helps you to be able to see yourself more clearly. While doing this, also take a look at the things that are present (or not present) in your life that positively affirm who you are. It could be spending time with girlfriends, going to church, taking walks, volunteering, or participating in hobbies. When you're single, claim your time to pour into yourself and develop your own interests. This is your chance to do *you*! It is easy to fall into the trap of believing that a partner will complete your life and bring you joy. But what are you doing, or could you be doing, on your own to foster your expansive wholeness?

While self-reflecting, ask yourself these three questions:

1. What aspects of myself do I feel good about?
2. What parts of my life fill me up?
3. How are the effects of historical or direct trauma showing up in me?

Question 1 will help you to identify your positive attributes, or *strengths*. Question 2 will uncover the spaces in which you feel *enriched*. Question 3 will help you to identify your vulnerabilities, or *hot spots*. By identifying these hot spots, which are rooted in past trauma, you are able to see when trauma shows up in the present.

When you take stock of how past trauma influences current behavior, you might discover trauma baggage that you are bringing to relationships. Sometimes, just sometimes, the age-old adage of "It's not them, it's you" is actually true. This is not to place blame, but rather to give you the freedom to see yourself clearly, without adding judgment. Your low self-esteem, trust issues, heightened sensitivity, anxiety, and inability to be vulnerable with your mate might actually be residue from past childhood abuse, parental loss, or intimate partner violence. This is where you pause and do the self-work so that you can start the process of healing before you enter into a relationship with someone else.

The trauma part is usually the hardest piece for people to identify, so let's take a closer look at how trauma can show up in relationships. Ask yourself these three questions:

1. How did I receive love from my caregivers?
2. What were my early models for intimate relationships?
3. What wounds do I still carry from childhood or past relationships?

If you grew up in a home where there was chaos, unpredictability, emotional volatility, or a lack of clear boundaries, these dynamics showing up in a present intimate relationship may cause some distress, but they will be familiar. If you experienced neglect, abuse, or exploitation, you may have developed a *trauma bond* with your caregiver that is replicated in adulthood with an intimate partner. When you experience abuse from a caregiver who also loves you, then you inadvertently learn to associate love with abuse.

Trauma bonding can develop in relationships where there are repeated cycles of abuse, devaluation, and positive reinforcement. Trauma bonds are the result of an unhealthy attachment. Children are attached to their parents, whom they depend on for many things, and an adult may be dependent on their partner for support or to fill emotional needs. The victim of abuse at first feels cared for, but over time this feeling is replaced with emotional, mental, and sometimes physical abuse. The trauma of abuse creates intense feelings that are difficult to understand because the abuse alternates with kindness. Victims realize the change has occurred but blame themselves for it and believe it's up to them to bring back the loving part of the relationship.

Here are some characteristics of trauma bonds with an intimate partner:

1. They are cyclical and depend on intermittent positive reinforcement.
2. You cling to the good days and use them as proof that your partner cares about you.
3. You trust your partner and hope to change him.
4. You protect him by keeping his abusive behavior a secret.
5. You justify or defend the abuse.
6. You create distance from people who are trying to help you.
7. There is a power imbalance whereby you feel that your partner controls you and you don't know how to resist or leave.
8. You are unhappy but still feel unable to end the relationship.
9. When you try to leave, you feel physically and emotionally distressed.
10. When you say you want to leave, your partner promises to change but makes no real effort to do so.

Trauma bonds can show up in adulthood as excessively focusing on the needs of the other person, trying to please that person in order to receive their love, pushing down your own feelings of anger or hurt, experiencing cycles of being rejected and then chosen again, and denying the validity of your own trauma-based anxiety. People with trauma bonds see themselves as "bad" and wish to be "good enough" to get the love and approval they desire from their partners. They are always trying to *prove* themselves.

When past trauma affects a present relationship, it can be hard to sort out what's coming from where. Let's take a look at three trauma-based thoughts and feelings that can happen in a relationship:

1. I feel rejected when my man says he needs some space.
2. I am afraid that he will leave me if we have a disagreement.
3. I feel insecure if he interacts with other attractive women.

To examine whether these fears are based in your present reality or your past experiences, write down the information that you have that supports your worry, as well as the evidence that goes against it.

As an example, let's look at #1: *I feel rejected when my man says he needs some space.* This feeling often stems from a fear of abandonment. So, look at the instances in which that fear showed up in your life and the evidence for and against your worry.

Evidence to support my worry:

**He went out with his friends one night instead of staying home with me.
He has been working longer hours.**

Evidence that contradicts my worry:

> He got us tickets for a play that I really wanted to see.
> He's been excited about our new home and brainstorm-
> ing decorating ideas.

When you do this, you might find that in fact there is not a pattern of rejection, but rather, your history of trauma has distorted how you see things.

It is necessary for you to resolve the trauma that can keep you un-knowingly clinging to the painful memories of the past, experiencing emotional suffering in the present, and stuck in a cycle of unhealthy behaviors. Past trauma can be a barrier to making healthy and lov-ing connections with people in the present. It can make it hard for you to see things clearly. However, when you become aware of these dysfunctional patterns, you are then able to gain control over your emotions and clearly assess what is happening in the relationship.

After you've done some self-work, think about what you want in a relationship. You should do this before you've even met some-one in order to prevent your memory from becoming fuzzy when you meet someone who's really "fine" but isn't looking for the same things in a relationship that you are. Whether you want just sex, ca-sual dating, an exclusive or open companionship, or marriage, iden-tify it. Then list the characteristics that are most important to you in a person. Be specific. Some common things that people name are spiritual, attractive, employed, and no baby momma drama. Or intelligent, has his own house and car, has good credit and no debt, comes from a good family, doesn't have children, has never been married, is successful and ambitious, has a sense of humor, is in good shape, and likes to travel.

Don't forget the red flags, or deal breakers, which might be things like a criminal record, substance use, lives at home, doesn't take care of his kids, is broke, or is in another relationship. When considering partners, always ask yourself what, if any, of your red flags are present. Engage in this process early, before becoming attached to someone, which makes it more difficult to walk away.

When you meet someone that you like, who has the same goals that you have, discuss expectations for the relationship early on. If you know that you ultimately want to get married and have children, does this person want that too? If you know that you enjoy being active, attending events, trying new restaurants, and doing outdoor activities, do you expect your partner to enjoy these things as well?

Discuss the large, overarching issues, such as who will be the primary earner (maybe both of you), how finances will be managed, whether you will have children and when, who will take on the bulk of the caregiving for the children (again, maybe both), how children from other relationships will be integrated into the family, and what role you will have caring for parents as they age. Also explore and discuss everyday things, like date nights; socializing with friends; the distribution of chores like cooking, cleaning, and running errands; and having time for yourself to sleep in or get your hair and nails done or work out.

Don't forget your emotional needs, such as feeling listened to, being supported, and receiving affection. Think about *your* needs. When we start dating, we can so easily slip into focusing on the needs of the other person and lose sight of ourselves. Be direct in asking for what you need and listen to the response. Often, women feel like their expectations should be self-explanatory. *I shouldn't have to ask for you to do something to make my birthday special. I shouldn't have to ask for you to comfort me when you see that I'm upset.* They falsely believe that their partner should be able to read their minds and know how to make them happy. In most cases, it doesn't work that way. They may also be afraid of being labeled as too needy or demanding or asking for too much. Be clear about what you want so you don't find yourself just going along with the get along so you can say you have somebody—and then end up unsatisfied.

Frustration comes quickly when partners' expectations are mis-aligned. When a relationship is on the rocks, a woman might bend over backwards to try to fix it. The relationship may be troubled because of broken trust, infidelity, addiction, financial problems, problems with intimacy or parenting, extended family drama, or communication issues. Whether it's through attempts to talk it out, buying gifts, planning vacations, or even suggesting therapy, you might find yourself pulling every trick out of the bag to avoid starting over or, worse, being alone again. In the process, you might be avoiding or denying the truth about the state of the relationship.

As strong Black women we are doers and fixers. This at times can lead us to falsely believe that we can fix everything—even things that are outside of our control, like other people's behavior. We tell ourselves, *If I keep showing him what a great woman I am, eventually things will get better*. Release yourself from the burden of blame for things not working out or the disproportionate responsibility of trying to fix it. Avoid staying too long in unsatisfying relationships thinking that things will change. When we sit around waiting for something to miraculously happen, we are relinquishing our power. We are holding on to a fantasy rather than accepting reality. Our power is in our ability to do what is in our control to make the best decision that we can, with the information that we have at that time, to take good care of ourselves.

Every one of us wants a solid relationship. But we often don't recognize what a strong relationship looks like. Healthy relationships have the following characteristics:

- Mutual respect
- Honesty
- Trust
- Empathy
- Boundaries
- Space for individuality
- Intimacy
- Open communication
- Support
- Safety

A healthy relationship is one in which you feel safe to be vulnerable and show up as your complete and authentic self. Resistance to vulnerability has kept strong Black women from being able to rest in the support and comfort of their partners. It has stopped us from being able to let go and trust someone else to take care of us for a change. But with the right ingredients in place, we can experience the joy of both giving and receiving love.

SIX

I Can Do Bad All by Myself

More than 40 percent of Black women experience intimate partner violence (IPV) during their lifetimes, compared with 31.5 percent of all women. *Intimate partner violence* is violence or aggression that occurs in a relationship between a current or former spouse or dating partner. It affects more than twelve million people each year and accounts for 22 percent of violent crimes against women.[1] It can include physical or sexual violence, psychological aggression, or stalking. Some of the more subtle forms of sexual IPV include pressuring you into having sex, ignoring your discomfort during sex, pressuring you to perform sexual acts that you are not comfortable with, taking intimate pictures without your consent, or removing a condom without your knowledge.

Younger women with low self-esteem, poor parenting, few friends, and a history of childhood maltreatment or delinquency are at greater risk for experiencing IPV. Other risk factors include economic stress, strained relationships with family, jealousy and possessiveness in the romantic relationship, and subscribing to traditional gender norms and gender inequality.

In 2013 the US Preventive Services Task Force recommended

that clinicians routinely screen women of childbearing age for IPV.[2] The task force is a group of national experts that makes evidence-based recommendations about clinical preventive services such as screening, counseling services, and preventive medications. Although its recommendations are widely accepted in the medical community, a 2002 study examining the rates of screening among family practitioners, gynecologists, and emergency room physicians found that only 6 percent of clinicians routinely screened their patients for IPV.[3] This failure to screen leaves many women without the information and resources that they need to take steps in order to keep themselves safe.

One of the defining characteristics of an abuser is superficial charm, such as excessive flattery, to lure in a victim. In the beginning, the relationship can feel like an intense and passionate whirlwind, as abusers tend to rush into things quickly, before you know much about them or their past. They use charm and other means to manipulate you, such as buying you expensive gifts and isolating you from friends and family. In order to reduce your power and independence, they may try to control your money by encouraging you not to work. Abusers have no regard for boundaries and may violate your privacy by calling at odd hours just to "check in" or showing up somewhere unannounced. The moods of abusers frequently shift. They are jealous and hypersensitive and blame you for their aggressive behavior. They often have a history of violent behavior, which they explain away by saying they are always provoked.

The *cycle of violence* includes four repeating stages:

1. **Tension building**—stress builds from day-to-day life; the abuser feels ignored, threatened, or angry; and the

victim is walking on eggshells, trying to be compliant and nurturing.

2. **Acute violence**—typically preceded by verbal abuse, there is an outburst of violence, and the victim feels powerless.

3. **Reconciliation**—the abuser feels remorse or fears that his partner will leave; he apologizes, displays affection, and promises to change; the victim wants to believe that the abuser will not be violent again.

4. **Calm (before the storm)**—the relationship is calm and peaceful. But intimate difficulties inevitably recur, leading back to the tension-building phase and starting the cycle again.

Short- and long-term physical problems associated with IPV include headaches, back pain, and gastrointestinal issues; mental health problems such as depression, anxiety, and drug or alcohol abuse; and life-threatening injuries that can even result in death. Unintended pregnancies can occur as a result of IPV through forced unprotected sex, risky sexual behavior associated with the abuse, or reproductive coercion that occurs when one partner interferes with the other's method of birth control. This is another way abusers try to control their victims and prevent them from leaving the relationship. Victims of IPV can be so fearful for their safety that they are unable to carry out day-to-day activities such as going to work, running errands, or socializing with friends.

The widespread problem of IPV, in general and especially in the Black community, is underappreciated. It is more palatable to accept the false narrative that IPV is a problem that affects others rather than the collective "us" as Black women, because in our minds we are strong and not susceptible to such vulnerability and weakness.

One example can highlight two common themes. In the fall of 2018, emergency room physician Dr. Tamara O'Neal was shot and killed by her ex-fiancé while at the hospital where she worked.[4] She had broken off her engagement weeks before, and her ex showed up at her job unannounced to demand his ring back. *Half of female homicide victims are killed by intimate partners, and 50 to 75 percent of domestic violence homicides happen at the point of separation.*[5]

In news coverage of the event, O'Neal was universally described as a beautiful, resilient, passionate doctor who had a deep faith in God. She was loved by many and had a strong support system, so everyone described their surprise at her tragic death. Some family members acknowledged that there had been a "disconnect" in the relationship with her ex, but no one thought she was in danger. It is unclear what, if anything, O'Neal shared with loved ones about her relationship or whether there were any unidentified warning signs. *It is not uncommon for women to hide abuse out of shame and embarrassment.*

The decision to end a violent relationship involves a complicated cognitive, emotional, and perhaps financial negotiation of disclosing, staying, or leaving. According to the National Domestic Violence Hotline, a woman will leave her abuser on average seven times before she leaves for good.[6] Women stay in abusive relationships for various reasons, including fear, intimidation, shame, being unable to support themselves independently, the possibility of homelessness, lack of family support, the welfare of children and child-custody concerns, and inadequate protection through the criminal justice system. Domestic violence is the leading cause of homelessness among women and children.

In an effort to protect the Black men in their lives, Black women victims of IPV may also be reluctant to turn men over to the criminal justice system, as they are already contending with day-to-day racism and discrimination. They also don't want to bring shame to their families and communities and are concerned that others will think negatively about them. This is yet another way in which strong Black women sacrifice their individual safety and wellness for the good of the community at large.

It often takes a personal experience with abuse to really understand how it can happen and how damaging it can be. In the third year of my clinical psychology doctoral program, even I was not immune to being lured into a relationship that was emotionally and verbally abusive.

When I met Nathan, I had been completely undone by a broken engagement and the unexpected end of a six-year relationship. Three months before the wedding date, seemingly out of nowhere, my fiancé had confessed that he thought that we should postpone the wedding. At first, I was in complete denial. I didn't believe him. But soon I realized that he was serious, and I felt persecuted and angry. *How could he do this to me and my family?* Then I started trying to *fix it*. I prayed, I went to church more often, I tried to reason with him. But he had put his stake into the ground, and I could do nothing to change his mind.

As I was facing the prospect of losing this relationship and my sense of self, my dad tried to console me. "Don't be weak," he told me. "Give him his ring back and be done with it." The message was *Hold your head up high and move on*.

Eventually, I ended up in total despair. I slept all the time and lost weight. I couldn't hear anything but the voices in my head replaying every conversation with my fiancé. I avoided interacting with people for fear that they would ask me something about my upcoming wedding. But at some point I started dated again, trying to fill the space and distract myself from my grief. Nothing really stuck, until I met Nathan.

For our first date, Nathan made a reservation at a quaint new Spanish restaurant. It was a snowy night in November, so he dropped me off at the front door of the restaurant as he searched for a parking spot. We sat across from each other at an intimate table under dim lights, and I smirked at his attempts to flatter me. He told me about his ambitious real estate business plans. He name-dropped the multimillion dollar firm that he was partnering with for the project. He looked deeply into my eyes and carefully selected his words. In retrospect, I believe he was studying me, my likes and dislikes, my insecurities and vulnerabilities. He was cool, and cocky, and though I was skeptical, I was curious enough to take the bait.

During the early months of our relationship, his garish charm, accompanied by expensive gifts and boasts of his accomplishments, distracted me from what later seemed shamefully obvious. I noticed the cracks in the façade but somehow had lost myself such that I trusted the fantasy rather than my own good sense. He had only a high school education and had never worked a traditional job, but he was adept at influencing people to buy in to his dreams.

His three-story townhouse, which I later heard he had acquired with the obligatory help of his last girlfriend, was an unfinished luxury rehab where knocks on the door from the sheriff holding eviction notices were regular occurrences. His business projects were funded exclusively by an esteemed group of people who were so eager to believe in the guaranteed tenfold return on their investments that they overlooked the failure of proceeds to materialize years after money had been exchanged and contracts signed. His relationships with friends and family seemed sparse and strained, exemplified by his grandmother asking me when I first met her, "What is a nice girl like you doing with this guy?"

But I wasn't the only one in the relationship dealing with the baggage of unresolved feelings of rejection and abandonment. I had attracted someone who shared the same wounds I had. Subconsciously, I must have thought that I could show him enough love, compassion, and acceptance to fix him, and in doing so, I would also heal my own childhood emotional wounds. Of course, it didn't work out that way.

Nathan told me that he had been physically and verbally abused by his father and stepmother when he was younger. He felt rejected and abandoned by his biological mother, who he said hadn't protected him from the abuse. Trying to conjure sympathy, he repeatedly told me, "I had two pairs of jeans, one pair of gym shoes, and slept on a mattress with the springs sticking out." He covered his wounds with anger and treated them with narcissism and materialism.

When Nathan's complete control over me was remotely threatened, he retaliated and defended his ego with the silent treatment and a disappearing act that conveniently afforded him the opportunity to entertain other women. This behavior was a trigger for my fear of rejection and abandonment, and in turn my trauma response was to try to make him come back.

The *silent treatment* is a passive-aggressive style of communication that people use when they become overwhelmed, angry, and frustrated and don't know how to express these feelings. It allows them to avoid conflict by shutting down emotionally, pushing feelings down, and not directly confronting issues. People pretend that they're "fine," don't care about the situation at hand, and are completely in control of their emotions.

When people give someone the silent treatment, they are often trying to punish the other person by making them feel the negative emotion (such as feeling hurt or rejected) that they feel. It can also be used as a manipulation, and when the silence is broken, the issue is swept under the rug and the problem is never addressed.

The silent treatment is a form of emotional abuse when intended to hurt you, take away your control, or silence you when you try to set a boundary. It can be used to shift blame onto you or make you feel guilty, and it ends only on the other person's terms.

Nathan used the silent treatment to regain his power and control and to punish me for causing him to feel hurt. It was also a way of displacing his anger onto me. *Projective identification* is a psychological theory that posits that a person in a close relationship, like a romantic relationship, can displace their feelings onto another, causing that person to feel what they are feeling. Indeed, I felt the anger, hurt, and rejection that Nathan felt.

Nathan's mood swings were dramatic, ranging from intense affection to anger, jealousy, and revenge, all of which I blamed myself for. I racked my brain trying to figure out what I had done wrong, until he returned with an apology and renewed romance. I inhaled these high moments, which became more fleeting and less satisfying over time, and minimized the lows. To prevent feathering him into a rage, I tiptoed around his fragile ego. He preyed on my desire for validation and manipulated me for money, the use of my car, and my expertise in writing intelligent-sounding emails.

Because we Black women can have a deep desire for love and companionship, we can be vulnerable to being taken advantage of. We might find ourselves doing favors, loaning money, providing sex, and taking care of things in exchange for what on the surface looks like a relationship. Eventually, it becomes apparent that our presence is only as good as what we can do for the other person, and always on their terms. When we need something, we're ghosted. We're doing all of the giving and not getting much back in return.

In my relationship with Nathan, my anxiety became debilitating, and I punished myself with self-deprecating thoughts. The hyperventilating, thumping heartbeat of anxiety, and heavy well of despair were in an intricate dance, and who was in the lead depended on the day. Questioning voices of blame, guilt, and self-doubt took over and kept me from being able to think about anything else. At the time, I didn't know how to take control of my thoughts, emotions, and behavior by reminding myself of my inherent worth and setting healthier boundaries. The world was acting on me, and there was nothing I could do about it. I felt powerless.

I hid the dysfunction and the effect that it was having on me as best as I could from my friends, who according to Nathan "weren't shit" anyway. They, in turn, protected my pride and privacy by turning the other cheek and not asking too many questions, but they held firmly to their disdain when I would scurry under another door of forgiveness.

For three and a half years, I kept riding the roller coaster of my emotions—frazzled and exhausted, but not quite ready to get off. I was chained to the recklessness of my capricious emotions, propelled by the view of myself through Nathan's eyes, and I selectively disregarded the rational information in front of me. I could see myself only in the diminished, not-quite-fly-enough, not-cool-enough, always-doing-something-wrong way that he saw me. I felt helpless and unable to make the situation better but nonetheless kept trying. Part of me maintained hope that things would miraculously get better, that one day he'd see the light and we'd live happily ever after. Another part of me desperately wished that some external force would act upon me and make me stop.

I should have known better, I told myself. *I should have known* that lying, cheating, and put-downs were clear signs that he didn't respect me. *I should have known* that I was being manipulated to do favors in order to garner his favor. *I should have known* that he was trying to control me with incessant phone calls and surprise visits and by keeping me away from my friends. *I should have known* that even though he said that he loved me, this was not love. *I should have known* that I couldn't fix him and that in fact it was my own suffering that needed the healing. That he couldn't make me see my own worth. That the affection that I thought I saw in those early weeks, that I was perpetually trying to reclaim, was all a ruse.

I should have known, but I didn't.

My relationship with Nathan prompted me to go to therapy for the first time. After two tumultuous years, it was becoming clear that I was in an unhealthy, emotionally abusive relationship, and I didn't understand why I was unable to simply walk away.

I got a referral to a therapist but still waited six months before calling to schedule an appointment. The idea of handling my brokenness in therapy seemed more burdensome than the shelter of avoidance. But I finally called and made an appointment.

"What's bringing you in?" the therapist asked me.

I replied brusquely, "I broke off my engagement." I pushed the words out before they got sucked back in.

My eyes instantly welled up with tears. Even though I was calling because I was beginning to see the destructive problems with Nathan, the engagement that had ended three years before had been the beginning of my downward spiral—so that's what I blurted out. During the first few sessions, I sat on the couch and selectively told my kind-eyed, messy-haired, middle-aged white woman therapist bits and pieces of the less shameful parts of myself. She spoke slowly, said *Ahhh* and *Mmm*, and asked questions without judgment that sought deep understanding. She wanted to explore the relationship model that had been set for me by my parents.

It was the first time I'd ever thought about how my relationship with my father affected my relationships with men—why I was beholden to their acceptance and approval and spun out by rejection. It was uncomfortable sitting on the other side of a couch, being examined. My parents didn't understand my need for therapy. They didn't see anything that was obviously "wrong." I was "fine."

Therapy gave me new insight into the origin of my emotionally driven, versus wise, behavior. The "wise mind" is a concept put forth by renowned psychologist Dr. Marsha Linehan to describe the place where the reasonable mind (where thoughts, decisions, and judgments are based on facts and rational thinking) and the emotional mind (where thoughts, decisions, and judgments are based on emotions or the way we feel) overlap to find truth and create peace.[7] In my search for a happy ending, I was grasping for the narrowly lost love of my ex-fiancé, the full acceptance of my father, and the belief that I was in fact *good enough*.

But it was still a while longer before I ended the relationship with Nathan. As I became more wise, my patterns, and Nathan's, became more clear to me. I understood why his emotional stonewalling, though distressing, was familiar. I established firmer boundaries and stopped taking on the emotional baggage that he tried to dump onto me. Therapy helped me to have a clearer view of myself, and I stopped seeing myself through his negative eyes.

With this new awareness, I was able to detach. With a renewed spirit, I intentionally placed things in my life that would bring me joy and allowed myself to enjoy them without fear of what he might do or say.

Therapy helped me to identify my vulnerabilities—fear of abandonment and rejection and desire for love and acceptance—and how my relationship behaviors were tied to my understanding of love, examples of intimate relationships, and early childhood wounds.

The first step to getting out of an unhealthy relationship where you experience emotional, sexual, or verbal abuse is to tell to a loved one or a mental health professional what you are going through. Even if you are not sure that what is happening is *really* abuse (this can happen when people are having mind tricks played on them), talk to someone. Maybe even stay with a friend for a few days while you collect your thoughts and develop a plan. Your abuser might be encouraging you to distance yourself from friends and family, or you might be doing so on your own out of shame or embarrassment, but lean into your support system.

If you are in immediate danger, call the police, go to a shelter, or both. Remember: You are not required to protect someone else's safety above your own. Don't pretend to be strong when you are legitimately in danger (even if you aren't admitting it to yourself). Being strong is getting the help that you need.

SEVEN

Suffering of the Womb

Research estimates that more than 80 percent of pregnant Black women have experienced a trauma and about 20 percent have a diagnosis of post-traumatic stress disorder (PTSD).[1] Pregnancy can worsen PTSD symptoms that already exist. Prepregnancy trauma (such as childhood abuse and intimate partner violence) is associated with poor pregnancy outcomes, including preterm birth, ectopic pregnancy, and spontaneous abortion.

Among people with a trauma history, the stress response system in the body can become overactivated, resulting in excess stress hormones (i.e., cortisol) being released into the bloodstream. This can lead to increased heart rate, high blood pressure, and negative birth outcomes.

In general, Black women are at higher risk for myriad reproductive health problems. We are twice as likely as white women to experience a miscarriage after ten weeks' gestational age, a late pregnancy loss, stillbirth, or infant death in the first year of life—all potentially life-threatening traumatic experiences.[2] Although Black women are twice as likely as white women to report high postpartum pain scores, we are less likely to receive prescription medication to manage the pain. Black women are three to four times as likely to die from pregnancy-related causes as white women.[3]

The myth that Black people are less susceptible to pain has prevailed in medicine for centuries. In the mid-1800s, the physician J. Marion Sims, "the father of modern gynecology," used enslaved Black women to develop and practice painful gynecological operations. More recently, research has shown that physicians are more likely to misdiagnose the pain of Black patients compared with white patients, and women compared with men. A survey of white medical students and residents found that the majority believed that Black people's nerve endings were less sensitive than white people's and that Black people felt less pain.[4] It seems that the idea that Black people are better able to handle suffering has bled into the medical community.

One particular problem that Black women face more than white women is uterine fibroids; Black women are two to three times more likely to have them than white women.[5] Uterine fibroids can be associated with an increased risk of infertility, problems with conception, spontaneous abortion, and various pregnancy complications. They also can cause a number of other health problems, including chronic heavy bleeding, anemia, urinary frequency, and pelvic and back pain. Black women tend to get fibroids at younger ages and experience more severe symptoms. They tend to wait longer to receive treatment for fibroids, which results in a hospitalization rate that is three times higher than that for white women. By age thirty-five, approximately 60 percent of Black women will have had fibroids.

Black women with a history of childhood physical or sexual abuse are at even greater risk for having uterine fibroids in adulthood.[6] Compared with those who report no abuse as children, women who have been abused are between 8 and 36 percent more likely to develop fibroids.[7] Children who have been sexually abused are more likely to be obese, which is also a risk factor for fibroids.[8] Additionally, traumatic stress affects the levels of the sex hormones estrogen and progesterone, which are thought to play a role in fibroid development and growth. The risk of fibroids increases with the length of time and severity of child abuse. Consistent and emotionally supportive relationships in childhood can buffer the negative effects of childhood abuse on adult fibroid risk.

In general, women who experience more stress are more likely to have fibroids, and the symptoms worsen as the stress increases.[9] Stress can lead to unhealthy behaviors such as physical inactivity, poor eating habits, cigarette smoking, and increased alcohol use, which may also increase fibroid development.

Fibroids contribute to a third of hysterectomies in the United States.[10] Black women are two to three times as likely as white women to have hysterectomies, a third of which are done in the peak childbearing years between ages eighteen and forty-five.[11] One of the major consequences of hysterectomies is that they eliminate a woman's ability to get pregnant, which can lead to feelings of grief and sadness. A hysterectomy can be especially traumatic for younger women, women who do not already have children, or those who were planning to have more children in the future. After a hysterectomy, women may worry that they have lost a part of their womanhood, will look less feminine, or will age more quickly, which can lead to depression.

The shame and embarrassment that women can feel over their inability to bear children are not experienced just by those who have had hysterectomies. And Black women, for whom caregiving and motherhood are parts of their core identity, can find it especially difficult if they are never able to conceive or carry a fetus to term. Those who have had repeated miscarriages may feel that their bodies are defective and wonder, *What's wrong with me?* If they become pregnant again, they can experience debilitating anxiety that they won't be able to sustain the pregnancy, which can increase the risk of preterm complications.

When my client Heaven arrived in my office for her first therapy session, she had been experiencing severe pelvic pain for months and was unable to have sex with her husband. She was referred to psychotherapy by a pain specialist. Her doctor thought that her symptoms were psychological rather than physical and were related to her history of childhood sexual abuse.

Roughly eighteen months before Heaven started therapy, she had undergone a procedure to have fibroids removed. About a week after the surgery, she went to an emergency room in an impoverished neighborhood of Chicago complaining of heavy bleeding and excruciating pelvic pain. She was told that this was normal, given her recent procedure, and was sent home. The way she was treated made Heaven feel invisible.

She endured the pain for a couple more weeks, and when it still didn't go away, she returned to the emergency room. This time she was examined, and it was discovered that the surgeon had left a metal clamp inside of her uterus. Still, without medication or intervention, Heaven was told to go back to the place where she had had the initial surgery for additional follow-up. She did that, and the clamp that had been inside of her for weeks was removed. But the bleeding and pain continued. A few months after the clamp was removed, her doctor told her that her persistent symptoms were caused by recurrent fibroids and recommended a hysterectomy.

Heaven was devastated. She and her husband were planning to

have a child together. Her husband didn't have any other children, and she felt it was her responsibility as his wife to give him a child. Heaven had been putting off the hysterectomy for months when she came to see me. She didn't want to let go of the idea of having another child, as she finally had a good man in her life.

During our session, Heaven repeated, "It just hurts so bad." She rocked herself back and forth with her arms wrapped tightly around her waist.

In addition to her physical pain, Heaven was also experiencing a ravaging depression. She confessed that she had not been this severely depressed since right after she gave birth to her daughter. She remembered feeling alone, sad, overwhelmed, and hopeless back then. She didn't think that she could handle the responsibility of her daughter and dropped her off at her mother's house. She disappeared with no contact for two weeks, until guilt drove her back home. During the time she was away, she realized that she didn't want to abandon her daughter, as she had been abandoned. Her desire to care for her daughter motivated her to get help for the depression. Heaven didn't recall whether she was screened for depression after giving birth, but she took the initiative to reach out to her Family Services caseworker to connect her to a therapist.

After years of feeling stable and in control of her life circumstances, Heaven found that the unexpected return of despair and hopelessness scared her and brought her back to therapy.

Let's return to my friend Nicole—who worked for the pharmaceutical company. Like Heaven, Nicole was also dismissed by the healthcare system, which put her life at risk. She had continued to excel in her career, was happily married, pregnant, and excited about starting a family. But she had experienced multiple adverse childhood events, including living in poverty, having a mother with a mental health condition and a problem with substance abuse, childhood sexual abuse, exposure to domestic violence between her grandparents, separation from her mother, and feelings of abandonment by her father. These traumas put her at risk for complications during pregnancy.

Indeed, Nicole's pregnancy was not without complication— she was diagnosed with gestational diabetes and preeclampsia. When she was six months pregnant, her blood pressure suddenly spiked while visiting family in the suburbs. She was more than an hour away from her regular healthcare provider, so she went to the nearest emergency room. When she walked in, the white male doctor looked right past her, as if she weren't there. "I felt dismissed," she said. "They saw me as just another person walking into a 'hood hospital." In a state of panic and disgust, she tried to leave the hospital, but her husband pleaded for her to stay. When she went back in, she was triaged in a dark and dingy hallway.

The doctor who had ignored her only moments before examined her and said, in a condescending and cavalier tone, "Okay, looks like we're taking the baby today."

"Wait, what?" Nicole said, knowing that this was not the news that she needed to hear, as she was only six months pregnant.

Nicole's fear intensified when he asked her, "If necessary, do you want us to try to save the baby or you?" and waited impatiently for her response.

Desperate for an alternative, Nicole called her regular ob/gyn, a Black woman. Her doctor encouraged her to stay at the hospital and tried to calm her down, but Nicole could hear the concern in her voice. For the next several hours, and into the night, Nicole used every fiber of her being to will her blood pressure down with the help of a hypertensive medication that she had been given. She slept in the emergency room overnight on a hard hospital bed with no pillows. She was discharged in the morning.

On the way home, Nicole called her doctor to let her know that she had been released. The doctor instructed her to go to her regular hospital immediately. Now that she was stabilized, the doctor told her that the things the other hospital had done were out of date and no longer a part of contemporary health care. When she arrived at her regular hospital, she was admitted and stayed there for more than a week. She spent the last seven weeks of her pregnancy on bed rest and delivered her daughter four weeks early.

The disparities in reproductive health experiences between Black and white women can be attributed to the sweeping effects of racism and discrimination. Black women with fewer years of education, less income, and no insurance have less access to high-quality health care. The health centers and hospitals in under-resourced Black neighborhoods often do not use the most current standards of care and technology. Whereas Nicole had the means to leave the community hospital and go somewhere else, many other Black women do not, and their differential outcomes reflect this fact.

Healthcare providers discriminate against patients on the basis of race and perceived social status, which can lead them to discount the experiences patients report and their preferences. Even Black women with means who receive health care in top-ranked institutions report that their expressed concerns are discounted and they receive substandard care that ultimately jeopardizes their health and the health of their baby. Furthermore, a recent study found that when Black babies are cared for by Black doctors after birth, their mortality rate is cut in half.[12]

My childhood friend Tiffany also experienced life-threatening pregnancy trauma, and even though she received her health care at one of the top-rated hospitals in Chicago, she unfortunately had a more grave outcome than Nicole. At twenty-five years old, she had a high-risk pregnancy with twins and was on bed rest for her last trimester. She spent the final month of her pregnancy in the hospital as she was dilated three centimeters and had to have a cervical cerclage to prevent late-term miscarriage or preterm birth. Her traumatic birth experience began when she noticed spots of blood on the bathroom floor. She immediately alerted the nurses, and they informed her that one of the babies' hands was sticking out of her vagina. She had an emergency C-section and delivered twin boys at twenty-five weeks.

During the delivery, both Tiffany's life and the lives of her babies were in danger. One of her sons, Jeremiah, was born weighing one pound, fourteen ounces. He had a cerebral hemorrhage and a heart murmur and required immediate surgery to close the hole that was in his heart. Given the severity of his medical condition, Tiffany's doctors gave her the option of attempting to save his life. Naturally, she asked them to fight to keep him alive. He remained in the NICU for three months. Jeremiah's twin brother, Aaron, lived six days before he died from maternal sepsis—a severe bacterial infection.

While Tiffany was in the hospital, her mother came to visit almost daily to offer support. Her boyfriend, the father of the twins, came only three times over the course of three months. He claimed he found it too difficult to be in hospitals and interact with a special-needs child. He gradually became more distant and didn't offer any financial or emotional support to her or their son.

When Tiffany returned home from the hospital with Jeremiah, she said that she was sad but not depressed. In the aftermath of a traumatic birth, and the death of Aaron, she also had to deal with relationship drama. Rather than get stuck in denial of what had already come to pass, she accepted the reality in front of her and focused her attention on how she was going to take care of business. Consumed as a first-time parent of a child with cerebral palsy, she had little time to slow down and attend to her feelings of grief. She stayed *strong*. She said, *I got over it and just did what I had to do*. She trusted in whatever God had in store for her.

Tiffany says that she is good at coping with hard times because, with kids, you have to be. When she's not driving her son to physical therapy or his other activities, she's planning family gatherings, attending church events, or planting vegetables in her garden. She relies on her mother and friends for support and is unabashed about saying exactly how she feels. Humor is her tool for communicating her true feelings. She makes single motherhood seem effortless.

But recently, she has found it more difficult to cope. As her traumas have accumulated—her best friend was shot and killed, and shortly thereafter she was robbed at gun-point while taking her children out of the car—her anxiety has worsened, and she has regular panic attacks. The panic can be triggered by something as small as running late, seeing men walking in the distance in her neighborhood, or hearing about violent events on the news. She is often in a state of worry and never knows when the next bad thing might happen.

Tiffany has sought out help to cope with all that she's been through. Her primary care doctor prescribed Xanax for her anxiety, and she takes it as needed. She also received a referral to see a therapist and attempted to make an appointment but was put off due to the long wait list—a common barrier that keeps people from getting the help that they need.

In recent years, pregnancy trauma and maternal mortality

among Black women has received increased attention. In 2018, tennis star Serena Williams's disclosure of postpartum health complications and accompanying depression highlighted the prevalence and severity of these issues among Black women and left many feeling disoriented. Williams had an emergency C-section, and the incision popped open because of intense coughing resulting from a pulmonary embolism. The doctors found a large blood clot in her abdomen. She had yet another surgery to prevent lung clots. Williams reports that she almost died.

After delivering her daughter, Williams spent six weeks in bed. She was overwhelmed and felt guilty about feeling sad about having a new baby—a common sentiment among women who are having a difficult time adjusting to motherhood. To imagine Serena Williams, the epitome of character strength and physical aptitude, compromised was unsettling to say the least.

Beyoncé has also spoken out about having a difficult pregnancy. While pregnant with her twins, she was diagnosed with preeclampsia and spent the last month of her pregnancy on bed rest. She delivered by emergency C-section because the health of her and her babies was in danger. The twins spent the first several weeks of their lives in intensive care. The experiences of Williams and Beyoncé let Black women know that if pregnancy trauma could happen to them, it could happen to anyone.

Approximately 15 percent of mothers experience *postpartum depression*, a change in mood that occurs during the first year after childbirth.[13] Symptoms include feeling sad, anxious, moody, irritable, overwhelmed, or fatigued or having frequent crying spells. They typically begin between a week to a month after delivery. Mothers with postpartum depression may have difficulty bonding with their babies, as feeling frustrated, overwhelmed, and irritable can make interacting with a baby challenging. In turn, they may avoid contact with the baby.

The demanding and unpredictable nature of caretaking a newborn can leave women feeling tearful, on edge, and defeated. This is especially true for those who are used to having everything under control in their lives. They worry that they will not be a good mother because things aren't coming as easily as they should. They can begin to resent their partner if a larger share of the caregiving duties are falling on themselves. Women with postpartum depression often feel guilty that they don't have the warm and fuzzy feelings they believe all new mothers have. If they took added steps to conceive, such as in vitro fertilization, they may regret their decision. In some cases, the symptoms of postpartum depression may be so severe that women have thoughts of harming themselves or the baby.

During this time, it is incredibly important for new mothers to let go of rigid expectations about what motherhood should look like, and what they should or should not be doing, and offer themselves grace and compassion. While schedules can help you stay organized, clinging to them too tightly can be anxiety provoking. Embracing the attitude of "good enough parenting" and allowing yourself the space to be imperfect can take the load off and help to ease the strain.

Postpartum depression differs from the "baby blues," in that the symptoms are more severe and last for a longer time. After childbirth, most women experience some measure of mood swings, irritability, feeling overwhelmed and anxious, and not feeling like taking care of themselves because they are so tired. But such baby blues, caused by postpartum hormonal changes, stress, social isolation, and sleep deprivation, tend to taper off by the end of the second week after delivery. Postpartum depression lingers.

Black women are twice as likely as white women to develop postpartum depression.[14] Women who have a history of depression, bipolar disorder, or trauma are also more vulnerable to developing it. Other risk factors include having a stressful life event during or shortly after giving birth, experiencing medical complications during childbirth, giving birth to a child with health problems, or lacking a strong support system. Women who have an unplanned or unwanted pregnancy, or problems in their relationship with their partner, are also more likely to develop postpartum depression.

The American College of Obstetricians and Gynecologists recommends that ob/gyns and other obstetric care providers screen patients at least once during the perinatal period (up to four weeks after birth) for depression and anxiety, with a standardized survey, and conduct a full assessment of mood during the postpartum period (up to one year after birth).[15] Women who screen positive should be referred to appropriate behavioral health treatment. However, this across-the-board recommendation does not more specifically address the fact that Black mothers are less likely to receive treatment for postpartum depression.[16]

Managing stress, including traumatic stress, by using healthy coping strategies is a critical first step that we as Black women must take in order to eliminate the racial disparities in maternal morbidity and mortality and infant outcomes. Although physicians are trained to have the expertise to provide you with essential health care, know that you are the expert of your own body. If you feel like something is wrong, trust your instincts and get a second or third or fourth opinion if necessary. Be an informed patient, doing research and being prepared with questions when you visit your doctor. Never be afraid to advocate for yourself.

PARENTING

"The fact that the adult American Negro female emerges a formidable character is often met with amazement, distaste and even belligerence. It is seldom accepted as an inevitable outcome of the struggle won by survivors and deserves respect if not enthusiastic acceptance."

MAYA ANGELOU, *I Know Why the Caged Bird Sings*

EIGHT

The Maternal Bond

Enslaved Black women lived in perpetual fear of being separated from their children if they, or their children, were sold. It is estimated that approximately one-third of enslaved children in Maryland and Virginia experienced family separation. The fear of separation haunted adults, who knew how likely it was to happen, and soon enough, naive children also learned the pain of separation.

Although the bond between an enslaved mother and daughter was the least likely to be disturbed through sale, owners could get large profits by selling pretty girls, especially light-skinned ones, into prostitution or concubinage. Enslaved mothers were also taken from their children to nurse the offspring of their masters, and enslaved children were torn from mothers and brought into the master's house to be raised alongside his sons and daughters.

The presence of mothers who had been separated from their spouse and orphaned children necessitated communal parenting. Children were cared for by "aunts" and "grannies" and other elder women who could no longer work. These extended families ensured that family members had their basic needs met but also provided them with emotional support. Today, Black women still depend on the support system of extended families that includes relatives and nonrelatives.

Separation can be traumatic for mother and child, no matter the reason—including young mothers being encouraged to give children to other family members, having too many other children to care for, leaving children with relatives while mothers set up a new life (as my grandmother did with my mother), or experiencing mental illness, substance abuse, or imprisonment. Even though the decision might be made with the presumed best interests of children in mind, it is still difficult and painful for everyone involved.

Let's return to Nicole. She was born to an unemployed, teenage mother in a small town in the rural Midwest. She never knew her father but fondly calls him a "rolling stone." She speaks loosely about the circumstances into which she was born and thwarts the potential for embarrassment with humor by saying, "My mother had me at fifteen, so what do you expect?" When Nicole was growing up, her mother suffered from mood swings, alcoholism, and an addiction to crack cocaine. Her family explained her mother's behavior by simply claiming *You know yo momma crazy*—as they hid their purses and wallets in Nicole's presence.

Nicole's mother's behavior was consistently erratic. She went from being the life of the party to being short-tempered and angry and refusing to talk to anyone. Nicole had to look for clues to determine her mood. On the good days her mother flitted from one thing to the next—photography, poetry, reading James Baldwin, or antique shopping. This is the mother whom Nicole looks back on fondly, the mother she longs for even today. Nicole knew her mother was having a bad day when she smelled bleach while her mother was on a cleaning fit, scrubbing down everything in the house. That was her cue to stay away.

When Nicole was born, her grandmother stepped in to help raise her, after she persuaded her daughter to not have an abortion. Mrs. Bea had moved to Michigan from Meadville, Pennsylvania, by way of Alabama. She had been sent to live with her grandparents in Alabama because her own teenage mother was pregnant again and could care for only one child. She had a high school education and worked for more than thirty years as an in-home caregiver. She was married for forty years to a janitor, and together they raised six children.

Mrs. Bea was a steadfast matriarch, provider, and caregiver for the family and was active in her community. No matter what her family did, she was there to support them and embraced them fully with forgiveness and compassion. For Nicole, she was a refuge from her mother's mental illness. Nicole admires her grandmother's strength, faithfulness, and unconditional love. She says she'll spend all her days trying to be like her.

Nicole's mother's mental illness left Nicole vulnerable to victimization. Maternal mental illness, like bipolar disorder, increases the risk for childhood maltreatment. Nicole's mother always needed a man around—men who vied for her mother's attention—and Nicole hated that. Then when she was ten years old, she was molested by her mother's husband. Nicole was confused about being touched by a man in a way that made her uncomfortable. She felt weird. She thought that she was smart enough to know that what was happening wasn't right, but she didn't know what to do to make it stop. So she blamed herself.

Although she didn't tell anyone what happened, she communicated her distress by acting out. She became more aggressive, got into fights, and was routinely kicked out of school. At home, she cussed out her mother and stepfather. At one point, she became so angry with her stepfather's presence in the house that she threw a lamp at his head.

Nicole didn't understand her mother's cycles of depressive loneliness and manic impulsivity and the way that she was ruled by her out-of-control moods. Her mother's mental illness clouded her judgment and her ability to make rational decisions, and it prevented her from being fully present for Nicole. So the summer after eighth grade, Nicole was sent to live with her aunt and uncle in Chicago. There, she was embedded in a supportive, stable, and structured family environment where her emotional and material needs were met. Her opportunity to thrive was further optimized as she was placed in a top-ranked high school where she excelled academically and flourished socially.

Despite her mother's challenges, Nicole knew that her mother loved her. When Nicole was a child, her mother told her every day that she was strong, smart, and beautiful. These words of affirmation nurtured Nicole's self-esteem and confidence through adulthood.

My client Gloria was separated from all four of her children when her ex-husband called Child Protective Services and reported neglect while she was at work and the children were with a neighborhood babysitter. Gloria had experienced sexual abuse as a child and domestic violence as an adult. Her motivation to escape the abuse at home, and deep desire for attention and affection, left her vulnerable to being lured in by a victimizer. Women who are sexually victimized during childhood or adolescence are twice as likely to be revictimized as adults.[1]

After Gloria married her husband when she was seventeen, he became more controlling and isolated her from friends and family. He put her down by telling her she was fat and ugly and convinced her that no one else wanted her. Sometimes, he didn't come home for days at a time, refused to tell her where he was, and had multiple relationships with other women.

When Gloria was eight months pregnant, her husband pushed her down the stairs and she miscarried what would have been their second child. He had complete control over the household finances, and she had no income of her own. She felt trapped. A few years later, after two more kids, he became so angry that he removed all of the appliances from the home, turned the heat and electricity off, and locked her out.

Gloria was now in the same situation in which her mother had been. As a child, Gloria had listened as her father told her mother, "You ain't shit, you stupid bitch," and watched with terror as his closed fist dislocated her mother's jaw and knocked her to the ground.

Without any other options, Gloria and her three children went to a homeless shelter. A few weeks later, when Gloria returned home, her mother moved in to try to help protect her from further abuse. She figured Gloria's husband would be less likely to abuse her if she were there. "That was Mom's way of making up for not protecting me from the abuse when I was younger," Gloria said.

For the most part, it worked, and the physical violence toward Gloria slowed down. However, there was an instance when Gloria's husband attacked her mother in response to getting involved in their business, and Gloria was left scrambling between them on the ground as she tried to pry them apart. Soon after, Gloria and her husband divorced. She and her children and mother moved out and got an apartment of their own.

The put-downs from Gloria's father and ex-husband played over and over in her head. She was passive, wanted desperately to be loved, and had difficulty establishing boundaries in her relationships. Burdened by feelings of rejection, she sought validation of her self-worth.

Eventually, she got involved with a friend of her ex-husband. In the beginning, while her mother was around, things seemed fine. He offered her the attention that she thought she needed. But after Gloria's mother died at age fifty-five, Gloria found herself vulnerable to victimization again. Her boyfriend's behavior started to change, and she discovered that he had schizophrenia. He heard voices, was paranoid, and acted violently and aggressively toward her. When the voices told him that she was cheating on him and out to get him, he screamed and lunged at her and tried to choke her.

Gloria's ex-husband was angry about the new relationship and became more so when Gloria and her boyfriend had a child together. Her ex-husband felt he had lost control of her and began to threaten and intimidate her. Gloria says her ex-husband's claims of child neglect were false and an act of revenge.

Gloria laments the separation from her children and believes that she did everything that she could to try to get them back. She complied with child welfare requirements to undergo a psychological evaluation, attended parenting classes, and had supervised visits, but to no avail. Of all the trauma that she experienced, the loss of her children seemed to affect her the most.

"My babies were taken from me and there was nothing that I could do," she told me with a tone of helplessness, checking to make sure that I was convinced that this was not her fault. She defends herself against the judgment that can come when mothers are not the primary caregivers of their children, no matter the circumstances.

Mental illness, drugs, and alcohol are usually the key culprits when children are removed from a home. In cases involving mental illness, even when women take the required steps to be unified with their children, they can ultimately be deemed unfit to care for them. They may have a subsequent mental break, receive inadequate treatment, not comply with treatment, or the treatment enables them to achieve only minimal functioning. Or they may simply fall through the cracks of the system.

The majority of children are taken from their parents' homes by Child Protective Services for allegations of neglect rather than abuse. Black women fear being reported to child welfare by neighbors, teachers, social workers, or police, who might judge them for the conditions of poverty in which they live and don't understand the decisions women need to make to care for their children. For example, a six-year-old child slips out of the house while Mom is taking a nap; an eight-year-old is left at home for thirty minutes while Mom runs to the corner store; a ten-year-old is given the keys and told to go straight home after school, approximately an hour before Mom gets home from work. The criminalization of parenting choices some poor women make has been dubbed "Jane Crow."[2]

The removal of children from their homes and placement into foster care can be traumatic. Children in foster care are four times more likely to be sexually abused than those who are not in care; the rates are even higher in nonfamilial foster homes and group homes.[3] Foster care can perpetuate the cycle of abuse because adolescent girls in foster care are twice as likely to become pregnant than their non-system involved peers.[4] Children who are born to teenage mothers are more likely to end up in foster care themselves. Adolescent mothers who give birth to their first child while in foster care are seven times more likely to have their child taken into custody before the child turns two years old.[5] In 2018 the Family First Prevention Services Act became federal law; it allows young women who become pregnant while in foster care to be eligible for up to twelve months of preventive services, including mental health, substance abuse, and parenting skills training intended to keep the mother and child together.[6]

Relationships with men, especially in situations where a spouse or boyfriend has caused harm to a child, can also play a role in the removal of children from their homes. These situations can become painfully complex when reunification between mother and child fails because the mother refuses to end the relationship with her man. She might feel like she is nothing without a man and in turn puts the needs of the man over those of her children. Alternatively, the mother might believe that since she wasn't mothered sufficiently, she can't be expected or required to give what she herself never received.

From an institutional perspective, child welfare caseworkers have the dual role of investigator and helper. Social service workers need to prioritize the safety of children, but heavy caseloads often mean that mothers do not get the services and support that they need. Additionally, some people in case manager and social worker positions don't have the adequate education, training, or compassion necessary to effectively carry out their jobs. These factors, coupled with racism, can prevent families from getting the full range of services that they require in order to care for their families and make better lives.

Gloria's children were placed in foster care with their paternal grandfather, where the cycle of abuse continued as he molested her two young daughters. She learned of this abuse years later when her daughters were adults, as she was still desperately trying to reestablish a relationship with them despite their disinterest. Gloria apologized to her children, but her apology was met with resentment.

They were angry that she had not been there to care for and protect them. Gloria didn't understand why they couldn't forgive and move on as she had done with her own mother.

My grandmother's courageous move from Montgomery to Chicago left my mother separated from her father, and temporarily, from her mother. On the way to Chicago my grandmother dropped off my eight-year-old mother at her baby sister and brother-in-law's house in Pennsylvania, while she went to get settled. My great aunt was married to a Baptist preacher with a penchant for chain smoking, whisky, and women. My grandmother never sat my mother down to tell her where she was going, or if or when she would be back. She just left. Likely, that was the only way that she could emotionally cope with being separated from her child.

Although some children who are suddenly and unexpectedly separated from their parents may experience the separation as traumatic or emotionally painful, my mother wasn't consciously aware of any distinctively negative feelings she had as a result of her mother's sudden departure. In fact, her memories about this period of time are sparse and shallow. I believe she may have distanced herself emotionally from the discomfort of these memories as a coping response, making it more difficult to recall specific details, as is known to occur among children who have been exposed to trauma.

Having a strong social support in place, such as extended family, can be critical in helping children cope with a parental separation. My mother was with her favorite aunt, in a safe and loving environment, where all of her needs were being met. After a year, my grandmother came back to get my mother and took her to Chicago.

The distance between my mother and her parents settled in a quiet and ordinary way. Although my mother didn't have the language to understand what was happening to her and my grandmother, and my grandmother did little to explain it to her, she does remember persistently feeling alone and unloved. The presence of her mother was empty, and her father was obscure.

In addition, an impenetrable emotional fortress surrounded my grandmother, and my mother was resigned to being unable to conquer it. Given little context with which to understand the way that Grandma interacted with her, she was left to create her own meaning. She surmised, *She just doesn't like me.* Grandma didn't read her bedtime stories, help with homework, shower her with hugs and kisses, or tell her *I love you.* Instead, she told her, "You just like yo daddy," the dead-beat whom my mother barely knew.

"It seemed like she was always mad at me," my mother said. She took her mother's sharpness personally and thought maybe it was her fault that she acted the way she did.

My grandmother was unable to relax into a soft, comforting love with my mother. But she gave her what she had, which was a dependable, hard-pushing, and protecting love. This love was designed to make my mother strong so that she could defend herself and would not be hurt by others, as she had been.

Black women's collectivist nature and the mentality that "it takes a village" to raise children are cultural strengths that we must continue to rely on to care for our families using all of the warm hands that we have available. We were not meant to raise children in isolation. Don't let shame of your individual family circumstance get in the way of your getting the support that you need to keep your family together, or enlisting another caregiver if that is the right decision for you. We must keep our children tightly knit in a community of love with their "othermothers" who are available to help keep them safe and provide counsel and wisdom.

NINE

Daddy Issues

A 2018 report showed that approximately 70 percent of Black children are born into single-mother households.[1] Even when children aren't born to single mothers, mothers may later become single because of parents choosing to no longer be involved with each other, incarceration, or death. Being born to a single mother doesn't necessarily mean that fathers are not present in the lives of children, as some "single" moms are unmarried but living or co-parenting with the father of their children or unmarried and co-parenting with the father. However, in cases where the father is absent, inconsistently present, or not helping with child support, children can have difficulty understanding the reasons for their father's absence and reconciling their feelings about it.

After my grandparents divorced, my grandfather quickly remarried and had six more children. In my mother's eyes, her father had abandoned her for his new family. She felt rejected. His new children had a father, and she didn't. She looked around at all of the other children in the neighborhood who had fathers and felt shamefully different. *Families are supposed to have a father*, she thought. *Why don't I have one? What's wrong with me?*

Psychologically, children who are suddenly separated from their parents can become emotionally numb and detached as a way of protecting themselves from the hurt of a future loss or disappointment. They seem unbothered and as if they don't care about much of anything.

My mother was apathetic when it came to her father. She didn't question his whereabouts or express feelings of longing for him. As a child, she saw him during occasional trips back to Montgomery to visit family. She felt odd because she felt no connection to him and didn't know what to say to him. "He was just somebody they told me was my father," she said.

When I was a little girl, I took a trip to Montgomery with my mother and visited my grandfather, who was living alone in the same house where he'd lived when he was married to my grandmother. At my grandmother's request, my mother drove my grandmother's big blue Cadillac and parked it in front of the dilapidated building on dusty gravel. We walked gingerly up the rickety wooden stairs. My grandfather opened the door smiling widely, eyes sparkling. The smile was familiar; it was my mother's smile, except that day, she wasn't smiling.

Grandpa was short in stature and stood hunched over, which made him look older than his years. He wore a wrinkled, dingy white T-shirt and jeans with brown dirt stains on the knees. When he invited us in, my eyes went straight to the kitchen sink full of dirty dishes and roaches crawling on the counters and walls. I scooched in closer to my mother on the old sunken couch that was covered by a sheet.

My grandfather sat kitty-corner from us in an armchair, leaning in toward us. My mother's empty eyes wandered, searching for something. When their eyes met, she snatched hers away. The three-blade window fan struggled to circulate the thick, muggy Alabama air. We talked politely for thirty minutes, he asked about my grandmother, and then we left.

My mother begrudgingly hosted him during his infrequent trips to Chicago. She tried to be strong and hide her frustration when he flashed his wide smile and politely requested that she run him to the liquor store "real quick" to pick up a pint of Crown Royal. In an effort to avoid conflict, she obliged, but she was annoyed. She didn't think that she cared whether or not he was there, but she also didn't want to push him farther away. The childhood feeling of helplessness returned, this time in her own home.

In 2001, when she learned of his death, she didn't show any emotion. She wasn't sure what to feel. At the behest of loved ones who thought she needed closure, she returned to Montgomery to attend the funeral of the father she barely knew. She was losing him for the final time. She and fewer than twenty friends and family sat in the barren funeral home in the country to pay their last respects. No one spoke or shared fond memories. Being the eldest child, she regrets not having spoken at his funeral. Today, his military flag sits on display folded in a glass case in the center of a bookcase in her home. After he had died, she said, "At least I knew where he was."

The family refrain of *At least I knew where he was* discounted any feelings that my mother might have had about not having a closer relationship with her father—because Black people's pain is always on a spectrum. There is always someone who has it worse off, and for that we should be grateful.

When I asked my mother how her early childhood experiences affected her, she paused and said, "I guess I never really thought about it." In the space between the question and the answer was a hint of sadness and concrete resistance to pain. My mother never thought of being separated from her parents as a child, growing up with an absent father, or living in poverty as being traumatic, and for her, maybe it wasn't. Under the shield of my grandmother, and other extended family, my mother emerged into adulthood with few wounds visible to the naked eye.

Just like my grandmother, my mother was rejected and discounted by a father who was only an arm's reach away. She was keenly aware: *this person is supposed to be here, but he's over there; he's supposed to care for me, but he doesn't seem to care.* And just like my grandmother, my mother never spoke of what it meant to her to not have a relationship with her father. She inherited not only the trauma but also the appearance of indifference and silence as a way of coping. His absence was never acknowledged. The space that he was supposed to fill was so fiercely guarded that it was rarely recognized that it even existed.

Children can feel a range of emotions in response to a separation or divorce. High levels of parental conflict during and after the divorce are associated with poorer adjustment in children.[2] The child may feel angry that their world is changing and they don't have any control over it. Without an explanation of what is happening, they may feel guilty and blame themselves. They can become anxious and worry that they too will be rejected or abandoned by one of their parents. Younger children may demonstrate separation anxiety—crying, clinginess, and frequently asking for the parent who is not around. The child's behaviors may change; they may begin to withdraw or have conduct problems, their academic performance may decline, and eating and sleeping patterns may change. They may choose a side and demonstrate preference for one parent and blame the other.

However, in general, children are resilient. Research has found that while divorce affects most children in the short term, they rapidly recover.[3] With a plan in place to help the child through the process, many of the potentially negative outcomes associated with divorce can be minimized. While this transition is happening, it is important to keep other aspects of the child's routine stable in order to provide them with a sense of security. Parents should let the child know what is happening, using language that they can understand, in advance of the actual separation. In these conversations, emphasize to the child that the separation is not their fault. Let other people in their life, like teachers, mentors, and friends know what is happening so that they can also offer support to the child. Give the child space for them to talk about their feelings openly and without defensiveness.

Just like my mother and grandmother, I too was raised by a single mother. Although my father was present, that presence had clear restrictions because I was never granted permission into his *other* life. My mother passed down to me her way of coping with our family arrangement, and any feelings that she may have had about it, by pretending that everything was "fine."

At home, the fullness of Mom's trustworthy presence filled in the spaces between Dad's comings and goings. Most of everyday life felt comfortably insignificant. In the mornings, there was just me and Mom in the house. Mom padded me with grits and sausage patties that stuck to my bones before sending me off to school with kisses on the cheek and well wishes for a good day. After school, she was waiting for me with a snack of graham crackers and sliced honey-dew melon.

When I played carefree outside with the four kids next door who had the *normal* family, Mom pulled the blue curtains back and watched me closely from the living room window. She was always checking for danger and making sure I was safe. She restlessly anticipated my comings and goings and any movement in between. I reliably felt the intensity of her protective covering. I took her tender, loving care for granted.

Before long, Dad came home. When I looked out of the backdoor window and saw the garage door rise and his car pull in, I was excited. I practiced my piano lessons and did homework at the dining room table while Mom made dinner and the six o'clock news played in the background.

The three of us settled into the easy warmth of the den. Dad stretched out on the couch with a beer in one hand and pipe in the other, Mom sat placidly in the recliner in the corner, and I sat on the floor and held the space between them. Some evenings I pulled out my chalkboard and taught them a math or vocabulary lesson that I'd learned in school that day.

My mother listened attentively and smiled approvingly. My dad, the educator assuming the role of the student, asked critical-thinking questions to test my comprehension. I searched the furrows of his bushy gray eyebrows and the corners of his mouth for the reward of his approval. And on Thursday nights, like most folks, we watched *The Cosby Show* and I dreamed of a family like the Huxtables.

As evening gave way to night, Dad asked me to get his shoes as he buttoned up his white dress shirt, tucked it back into his pants, and placed his tie back around his neck. This was the signal that he was preparing to leave, to return to his "real" home with his wife and child—something I didn't realize in those early days. Family time was over.

Every night for a long time it was the same. "Daddy, where are you going?" I'd ask. "To see a man about a mule," he'd reply.

At first, I was amused by his mysterious response. I accepted it eagerly as a riddle that I was smart enough to solve. As I got older, I became angry that my inquiry was so easily dismissed with laughter or silence, deemed unworthy of a true response. Desperate for him to stay, I wrapped my slight body tightly around his legs. He labored toward the door, dragging me across the carpet as I sat on his feet and refused to let go. When my pleas failed, I begged him to take me with him.

Sometimes my mother said sarcastically, "Why don't you take her with you?" It was a thinly veiled threat intended to test his allegiance. Her anguish appeared only briefly before her aversion to conflict swept it away.

Once, at the peak of my protest, I declared, "Fine, then I'm leaving and I'm not coming back!" I was certain that this would usher him to his senses. I packed my little pink square suitcase and marched confidently out of the house and down the block to the park where I sat on a bench and waited for someone to come and get me. No one did.

After about thirty minutes, I walked back home, sullen and defeated. I was frantically trying to outsmart the end of Dad's presence, and when my efforts failed, I felt rejected. He left without looking back, and Mom turned the lock on the door behind him. My eyes clung to the backdoor window as he backed his car out of the garage and drove away.

I simultaneously felt the love and safety of a "normal" family and shamefully different. While my mother's default position was to uphold the tradition of silence and convince herself that everything was "fine," my desperation for the relief of answers wouldn't allow her to do so. Combined with my genetic predisposition for traumatic stress, the felt abnormality of my home environment made me anxious and depressed. I bottled in the nervous energy of our family secret without ever being explicitly told to do so.

My unrelenting questions forced my mother to confront that which she would have preferred to sweep under the rug. Backed into a corner, she made a good-faith attempt to explain our unconventional family structure to me using Barbie dolls. She pointed to her and me in the doll house and then put Ken in the pink Barbie Corvette and drove him away. "This is your dad going to his other family's house," she said. The unsatisfactory explanation brought more angst and uncertainty. As the veil over my decidedly shameful home environment was raised, I became more rebellious and angry by my dad's partial presence and apparent disregard for the feelings of me and my mother.

My home life didn't match my understanding of what a "normal" family was supposed to look like. I imagined what these other people whom my dad lived with must be like, living in their fantastical house in the suburbs with their Lassie dog. I didn't understand why I wasn't allowed to go there with him. Occasionally I would call on the phone, and when I'd hear a lady's voice answer, I'd hang up.

I didn't know where I fit in this picture. My mind raced with questions. Dad was fully embedded in our family, but we were only a fraction of his. Just as it had been with my grandmother's father, and my mother's father, my mother was in the background of the family that my dad claimed.

With every reach for full entry into my father's life that was returned empty-handed, I ached. My need for validation was burgeoning, ready to be filled by him or another. I tried earning his approval by chasing achievement, which I believed would ultimately persuade him that I was good enough for him to want to stay. But with him, there was no such thing as good enough. As soon as I met the bar, it was raised. Praise was hard, if not impossible, to come by, yet I craved it no less. I cycled through loops of intense admiration and idealization to righteous indignation. For months I gave him the silent treatment, passive-aggressively creating a boundary, the same way he did with me and my mother.

Love and rejection were inextricably intertwined. When I was blown back by rejection from my father, I fell into my mother for comfort. She was a steady and reliable mainstay. From her perspective, all of our needs were met. She had a secure job, a comfortable and safe house, a reliable car, a few dollars to do nice things. I had a father who was mostly present, which was more than she'd ever known. Any emotional needs she might have had were rendered insignificant.

The absence of her father and the coldness of her mother shifted her perspective in ways that she was unaware of. She was too proud and self-sufficient to ask for more than was voluntarily given. While she suppressed her emotional discord, I proclaimed mine freely. My loud and tangible feelings fanned the flames on hers. When I cried, the clouds in her eyes darkened. Her pain shown through mine reflected back to me. But she didn't know how to have a conversation about feelings or how to respond in turn. She'd tell me, "You need to calm yourself down." We both needed to be strong and in control.

Over time, the cycle of coming and going, dependence and rejection, developed my anxious-preoccupied attachment style. Adults are described as having four main styles of attachment, one secure and three insecure (anxious-preoccupied, dismissive-avoidant, and fearful-avoidant), that are developed as a result of interactions between children and their caregivers. These styles affect relationship functioning in adulthood. The anxiety that I felt in response to the variable presence and approval of my father when I was a child showed up later in my romantic relationships when I was an adult.

Similar to children of divorce, children who are born of infidelity also experience an intense range of emotions. They can be frightened and anxious, feel rejected, and feel as if they have done something wrong. These children often sense when a parent is spending time and emotional energy outside of the family and feel angry, betrayed, and embarrassed that the parent has chosen someone else over them.

Children may be put in a position where they are not only told to keep the secret of the infidelity, but also become the secret themselves, leading them to feel like the family "black sheep." Surely I felt this way when I was kept away from my dad's side of the family, not invited to family gatherings, and only acknowledged as his daughter to a select few in the circle of trust. Children in these situations are often faced with two choices: (1) accept the unacceptable—that they have been betrayed by the parent and hope that by keeping the secret they will receive the parent's love and affection, or (2) express outrage and risk being abandoned by the person whose love they desperately want and need. They are in a lose-lose situation. Over the years, I flip-flopped between both of these options.

Children born to infidelity often grow up to have difficulty in their own intimate relationships. They lack confidence in themselves, have a hard time trusting others, and have low expectations for their relationships. Sometimes, they repeat the infidelity that was modeled to them.

Our childhood experiences at home lay the foundation for

how we see the world. They establish what is "normal," how we relate to others, and how we see ourselves. Home is where we witness our first model for intimate relationships—our parents. The formative experiences of a child are directly affected by the experiences of their caregivers.

As children transition into adolescence and adulthood, they come to see themselves as unique individuals who exist within a larger system of family, community, and society. They develop beliefs about the circumstances in their environment that are in their control versus out of their control and what they have the power to change as opposed to what they must merely deal with. Through this positioning in multiple intersecting spaces, they develop a felt sense of where they are accepted and belong versus where they are rejected and don't fit. The parental relationship (no matter what it is) will set the stage for our intimate relationships down the line.

Breaking the cycle of splintered families is difficult, if not impossible, to do without first addressing the role that intergenerational trauma plays in our intimate relationships and parent-child relationships. We must cultivate awareness of unhealthy relationship patterns that are symptoms of unaddressed trauma in order to prevent repeating these cycles. Secrecy, denial, and avoidance keep us stuck in suffering.

VULNER-
ABILITY

somebody/ anybody
sing a black girl's song
bring her out
to know herself
to know you
but sing her rhythms
carin/ struggle/ hard times
sing her song of life
she's been dead so long
closed in silence so long
she doesn't know the sound
of her own voice
her infinite beauty
she's half-notes scattered
without rhythm/ no tune
sing her sighs
sing the song of her possibilities
sing a righteous gospel
let her be born
let her be born
& handled warmly.

NTOZAKE SHANGE, *For Colored Girls Who Have
Considered Suicide When the Rainbow Is Enuf*

TEN

The Buildup

As we have seen, childhood traumatic experiences can affect mental and physical health in adulthood. Children who have experienced a traumatic event are more likely to become adults who have chronic disease and mental illness, abuse drugs and alcohol, and are the victims of violence. They may also have difficulty with psychological adjustment in that they experience guilt, feel insecure, fear abandonment and rejection, have difficulty forming secure relationships, and struggle to function at home, school, and work. However, the myriad challenges that Black women face in adulthood are often disconnected from their early childhood experiences. Indeed, familial, environmental, and situational factors, and the availability of support, all contribute to the impact that trauma can have over the course of a Black woman's life.

I first met my friend Amber at a cocktail reception for an executive education program. This former beauty pageant queen stood out from the crowd, wearing a yellow dress in a room full of black and gray suits. She walked around the room confidently, unafraid to make her presence known. You wouldn't have guessed that she had endured multiple traumatic experiences during her childhood that slowly but surely started to affect her mental health as an adult.

When Amber was in the sixth grade, her mother had a nervous breakdown. She had severe panic attacks, stopped eating, and did not come out of her room for days. Eventually, she was hospitalized after being diagnosed with bipolar disorder, also known as manic-depression, and severe depression. Amber's mother also had a history of childhood sexual abuse, as she had been molested by an uncle. On good days, she was happy and excited about life and engaged with Amber and her siblings, reading and playing. On bad days, she was angry, lashed out, and cried a lot.

Amber never knew which day was going to be which, but she always knew when her mother was raging. She and her siblings could never be still or quiet enough. They couldn't breathe without her becoming upset. Sometimes Amber and her younger sister had to bathe their mother because she was so depressed that she couldn't get out of bed. During these times, they made special efforts to be quiet and stay away from her—and, preferably, get out of the house.

Psychologist Lynne McCormack has found that children of a parent with mental illness often feel invisible and helpless.[1] Because their home environment is unpredictable, they can be anxious, filled with uncertainty, and have a heightened alertness regarding their surroundings. They are never sure what mood they will be met with and what the next day, or even the next moment, will bring.

These children often feel as if they have to compete with their parent's illness in order to receive the attention and care that they need. The "manic" symptoms of bipolar disorder—euphoria, aggressiveness, impulsively getting into relationships, instability at work, spontaneously leaving town—prevail and leave the child neglected. The dysfunction that children experience at home leads them to feel lonely, different, and stigmatized in relation to their peers.

Children of parents with mental illness often have to care for their parent—running errands, feeding and bathing them, or stepping up to care for younger siblings—as Amber did. These children grow up fast and learn quickly that in order to survive they have to figure out how to take care of themselves. To keep the peace at home, these children may try to soothe the sad and depressed parent, calm down the angry parent, or play intermediary between the parent and other people, such as family members or teachers. To try to gain some stability over their environment, they become skilled negotiators and are extremely perceptive and adaptable.

After Amber's mother was discharged from the hospital, she refused to take medication or receive ongoing outpatient mental health treatment. She didn't want to talk to anyone about her diagnosis because she thought that it meant that she was weak, crazy, and unable to function. She rarely went outside and didn't let people come into the house. Amber and her siblings were forbidden from talking with people outside of the family about what was going on at home. Amber felt trapped.

Amber's grandmother, Mrs. Mary, lived with her and filled in where her mom was unable to be present. Whenever her mom had an "episode," her grandmother would say, "Mom isn't feeling well" or "Mom is having a bad day," but she never explained the nature of her illness. She took Amber and her siblings to their doctors' appointments, registered them in school, attended parent-teacher conferences, picked up report cards, and attended recitals, award shows, and other activities. Amber relied on her grandmother for everything. She was the rock of the family.

In Black families, even when we know that there is a mental health issue, we can be slow to seek professional treatment. These are the types of problems that are best treated in the privacy of our own homes. We fear the consequences of adding yet another stigmatizing label to a person and don't trust systems that perpetually disenfranchise us. In our eyes, "telling" on a family member would surely make things worse—when in fact telling is the thing that could prevent the mental health issue from getting worse and becoming a downward spiral.

Amber's grandmother also suffered from untreated trauma and mental illness, and while she was caring for Amber, she was enveloped in her own emotional pain. She'd had nine miscarriages before Amber's mother was born. She'd also had a strained relationship with her own mother, who was deceased, and had hallucinations that her mother was coming into the house and leaving notes, as if she were still alive. Amber's grandmother blamed herself for the sexual abuse that her daughter had endured, and the accompanying depression, and punished herself with the thought that she should have known and protected her.

Amber felt ostracized and believed that other people didn't have these types of problems. On top of everything else, when she was in eighth grade, her house burned down when three Molotov cocktails were thrown through the front door window. Her family had received a series of racist threats and bricks had been thrown through the window because the neighbors did not want Black people in the neighborhood. After her family lost their home, Amber and her mother, grandmother, and three siblings moved into a one-bedroom apartment with her grandfather. In this small space she was in even closer proximity to her mother's mental illness.

Amber's genetic vulnerability to mental illness, combined with the stress and trauma of her home environment, made her more vulnerable to depression and anxiety. She felt lonely because she didn't have anyone to talk to about what she was going through. She didn't have many friends and was bullied at school because she couldn't afford the things that other kids had. She felt like she could do nothing to change her situation.

But the one thing that Amber *could* control was food, so she stopped eating. In addition to the depression and anxiety, she developed anorexia, an eating disorder whereby a person has an extreme fear of gaining weight and restricts the amount of food that they eat, and in turn becomes severely underweight. People who are anorexic use food to cope with the emotional distress caused by a chaotic, unpredictable home environment. Eating disorders like anorexia often go undetected in Black women because excessively restricting food and watching one's weight are mistakenly labeled as being healthy.

We accept the stereotype that Black women don't have mental health problems and certainly not eating disorders. Although anorexia occurs at lower rates in Black women than white women, binge eating, whereby a person consumes unusually large amounts of food and feels unable to stop eating, occurs at higher rates in Black women than white women.[2] It is an attempt to control what feels out of control in one's life.

As Amber grew into adolescence, her suffering increased. But her mother discouraged her from getting mental health treatment. "Don't go telling those white people our business," she said. Amber also wasn't convinced that talking to someone would solve the issues that were going on at home, stop the bullying at school, or make her feel better. She said the only thing that saved her was that she didn't like seeing her mother hurt. She wanted her mom's approval on everything, so she pushed through, continuing to be a "good girl" and help the family even when she was dealing with her own emotional pain.

Like a strong Black woman, Amber coped by taking control of everything that she could. She balanced being in high school, applying to college, and taking care of her siblings. When Amber was in eleventh grade, her mother was falsely accused of a crime and incarcerated. She was held on a bail that the family could not afford. People with mental illness are disproportionately represented in jail, where they are less likely to get the mental and physical health treatment that they need. While in jail she was diagnosed with stage-4 colon cancer.

Six months into her mother's incarceration, Amber adopted her two younger brothers. She didn't want to risk her and her brothers being split up and going into the foster care system. Amber's mother was incarcerated for more than two years, until she died.

Amber tried a few sessions of therapy in college after her mother died, but she didn't feel like the old white male therapist whom she saw truly understood her. He seemed to be just doing his job. She dropped out and continued trying to manage her feelings on her own.

After Amber's mother died, her grandmother's mental health rapidly deteriorated. At night, she believed that people were coming into the house and stealing things. The house was under lock and key, with several home security services, but she still worried that people were out to get her and her family. She stopped eating for days and threw things out of the fridge for fear that they were being poisoned. She stopped taking care of herself and could no longer live independently. Extended family explained away her delusions and hallucinations as just the way that she dealt with grief.

In some way, having the responsibility to care for her daughter had given her a sense of purpose and kept her well. After her daughter died, she gave up. Many years later she was diagnosed with paranoid schizophrenia.

Now Amber holds her grandmother's power of attorney and manages all of her affairs. Sometimes she feels overwhelmed, but she doesn't believe she has a choice other than to stay strong, push her feelings aside, and keep going.

Black adults with mental health needs are 50 percent less likely than white adults to receive treatment. Many Black women do not seek mental health treatment because of myriad barriers, such as not having mental health benefits as a part of their health insurance and expensive co-pays or out-of-pocket costs.[3] They may not be able to find a mental health provider who meets their preferences (race, age, gender, religious background). There may not be any providers who are easily accessible in the neighborhood, and if there are, they may have long waiting lists or may not be accepting new clients. If a person finds a provider, they may feel that they don't have the time or emotional energy to attend sessions. Childcare and/or transportation can also pose additional challenges.[4]

Black women often express their preference for a Black woman mental health provider—of which there are few. We want to be able to talk to a therapist with the casualness of a friend but receive the advice of a professional. We believe that a Black woman will be more likely to understand our struggles and less likely to judge us. When a client gives me the *You know what I mean, girl* eye, I smile and nod, and they know that *I get it*.

We as Black women want our therapist to have a basic working knowledge of our lived experience with racism and sexism without having to explain it. We want to come in as we are and don't want to feel like we have to code-switch in order to save face in front of a white person who we fear might minimize or stereotype us if we talk bluntly about our issues. We want someone who intimately knows (and loves) our culture, its strengths, and its vulnerabilities.

Like Amber, when things started to pile up for Nicole, she reached out for therapy but dropped out after the first session. After Nicole gave birth, her stress, anxiety, and panic skyrocketed. Having a daughter triggered memories of being victimized as a child. She worried relentlessly about her daughter's safety, guarding her closely and rarely letting her out of her sight. She admitted that she was paranoid and saw almost everyone as a potential threat, but she couldn't let herself give in to reason. Because she trusted so few people, she shut herself off from the support that was available and rarely had time for a break.

Nicole had dealt with her early childhood trauma and provider and caregiver stress by avoiding thinking about it and burying the feelings of distress. She realized that she probably needed to attend to these thoughts and feelings because she suspected that they were having an impact on her life in the present. But these life experiences, combined with her mother's mental illness, predisposed her to depression and anxiety.

Despite her attempts to avoid and deny, sadness, anxiety, and panic kept rising to the surface. She was ambivalent about seeking mental health treatment. Occasionally, she considered going to therapy, but she felt that seeing a therapist was just one more thing she didn't have time for. She reasoned that she was "fine" and could cope with her feelings on her own.

Six months after her daughter was born, the uncle who had taken her in unexpectedly died of a heart attack. "I've never felt more broken, lost, and unable to cope with what was in front of me," she said. "I didn't know if I would ever feel normal again."

Nicole was blown back by something out of her control—a traumatic loss. The person who had protected and provided for her was gone, and her sense of safety and security was destroyed. She was plagued by worry about her health, safety, and well-being and that of her family—the people she cherished most. It was difficult for her to see a way out of the grief. These feelings lasted for months without letting up. She felt as if her entire world was falling apart.

In addition to her mental state, her physical health began to decline. As her panic attacks became more frequent, her blood pressure skyrocketed. She gained thirty pounds and was diagnosed with type-2 diabetes. The fact that no one around her seemed to understand the deep despair she was experiencing made her feel more helpless and alone.

Nicole's optimism about being able to fix things on her own started to wane, so she contacted a therapist. But even after she identified the need for therapy, she delayed seeking treatment because she was overwhelmed by the process of choosing someone. She was daunted by the thought of just selecting someone from the Yellow Pages with whom she would share her whole life. Ultimately, her primary care doctor referred her to a thirty-year-old, fresh-out-of-graduate-school, perky white female clinical psychologist. Nicole was skeptical about going to see this therapist because she didn't think there was any way that this younger white woman would understand the challenges that Nicole faced as a Black woman.

At the first visit, the psychologist recommended that Nicole start group therapy. This instantly put Nicole off and shut her down. She was leery of therapy as it was, and group therapy was not even a consideration. She couldn't imagine sharing her most intimate secrets with a group of troubled strangers. The therapist did not offer a treatment plan that felt acceptable, so Nicole stopped therapy before barely even starting.

When Black women receive care from non-Black providers, they may not receive culturally competent mental health care—treatment that includes foundational cultural knowledge and adapts to the cultural contexts of the individuals whom they serve. This can lead to premature disengagement from treatment. For example, Black women may have a therapist who does not understand their historical trauma, the cultural expectation to be a strong Black woman, the role of spirituality in healing, or the fact that Black culture is more collectivist than individualist.

Indeed, research has found that when the race of the client and mental health provider are matched, the client is more likely to stay engaged in treatment and has better long-term outcomes.[5] However, not many Black mental health providers are available. According to the American Psychological Association, in 2015, only 4 percent of psychologists in the United States were Black.[6]

When Black adults do receive mental health treatment (such as medication or psychotherapy), they are more likely to receive it from a general medical provider such as an internist versus a mental health specialist.[7] Mental health treatment within the primary care setting can feel less stigmatizing than going to a psychiatrist (a medical doctor who prescribes medication) or a psychologist (PhD or PsyD who provides talk therapy, or cognitive and behavioral interventions).

In January 2016 the US Preventive Services Task Force issued a recommendation that all adults be screened for depression in primary care.[8] The Affordable Care Act (ACA) expanded coverage for mental health services; depression, alcohol misuse, and domestic violence screenings are considered essential health benefits that must be covered in new health plans.[9] Depression screening is commonly conducted using a brief questionnaire that is administered by a physician's assistant or nurse and asks questions such as "Do you feel down, depressed, or hopeless?" "Do you have trouble concentrating on things such as reading the newspaper or watching television?" and "Do you have little interest or pleasure in doing things?" Note: your doctor should be asking you these questions at every annual visit.

A national study found that in 2012 and 2013 less than 5 percent of adults in primary care settings were being screened for depression.[10] Black people were half as likely as whites to be screened, and older adults were half as likely as middle-aged adults to be screened. The study found that Black and older adults often exhibited the physical symptoms of depression, such as headaches, body aches, and fatigue, rather than the mood symptoms, such as feeling down or sad. This made the depression more difficult to recognize.

People who screen positive for depression during a regular healthcare visit are either treated directly by their primary care provider or referred to a mental health specialist. In primary care, antidepressants are the most commonly offered depression treatment.[11] However, Black adults are less likely than whites to find antidepressants acceptable and are less likely to take them as prescribed.[12] It is not unusual for someone to receive a prescription for a medication and to never fill it. Alternatively, they may take a medication for a few days and then stop before it has had a chance to work, or they may take the medication "as needed," which is also ineffective. It can take two to four weeks for antidepressants to start working and up to eight weeks for them to reach maximum efficacy. Furthermore, people may have negative attitudes toward medications, such as the belief that the medications are addictive and concerns about side effects (such as "becoming a zombie," gaining weight, or losing their sex drive), or they may assume that the medications will not work.

New clients often tell me at their initial therapy appointment that they do not want to take medication for their mood. After letting them know that I understand and respect their preferences, I explain that it is my job to assess the information that they share with me and offer them the most appropriate treatment plan. I ask whether it will be okay to discuss the possibility of medication at a later date, if necessary, depending on what we uncover over the next several weeks. They almost always say *Yes*.

Psychotherapy alone can effectively help many individuals learn skills to resolve their stress, depression, and anxiety. However, other people may have more severe symptoms that are better treated with a combination of medication and therapy. If, after a few weeks of working with a client in therapy, I find that their symptoms indicate they would benefit from a medication evaluation, I refer them to a psychiatrist. I underscore that this referral is an opportunity for them to gain information on how medications might help them.

Similar to what can happen in primary care, some people fill the prescription and never take the medication or stop taking the medications because they don't immediately notice an effect. But others take the medication as prescribed, start to feel better, and wonder why they didn't take medications sooner. Medication can help a client to get out of the fog of suffering such that therapy is more productive and effective.

People who have other chronic health conditions, such as high blood pressure and diabetes, often think that taking medications for their *physical* health is a higher priority than taking them for their *mental* health. Yet people with untreated depression are less likely to adhere to the medications they take for their physical health. While primary care providers are an important resource for screening and providing medication treatment for people with mild symptoms of depression or anxiety, often triggered by an acute stressor (such as difficulties at work or grief), they have less specialized training in helping people with more complex backgrounds, such as someone with a history of trauma and multiple social and environmental stressors. Typically, primary care providers see their patients only briefly, one to two times a year, and do not have the capacity to offer them ongoing therapy.

Black people who do receive mental health treatment are less likely to receive minimally adequate care, considered to be a minimum of four sessions of therapy within twelve weeks of first depression diagnosis or filling a prescription for antidepressant medication for 84 of the first 114 days of treatment.[13] People often drop out of therapy prematurely after attending only a few sessions. Someone might attend sporadically, frequently canceling and rescheduling appointments, such that they never form a strong therapeutic relationship. In these cases, therapists are unable to develop a consistent relationship and comprehensive picture of the struggles clients are facing and in turn are limited in the support that they can provide. Delaying or discontinuing treatment increases the likelihood that symptoms will persist and become more severe, as will associated problems such as difficulties at school, at work, with family members, and in relationships.

On top of all of that, Black people are less likely to trust medical professionals in general. Our concerns, which have merit, are associated with potential consequences of seeking treatment that include loss of confidentiality, involuntary hospitalization, and involvement with the child welfare or criminal justice system. This mistrust of the healthcare system is in part historically rooted in the Tuskegee Study of Untreated Syphilis in the Negro Male conducted between 1932 and 1972 by the US Public Health Service.[14] The six hundred men who participated in the study were never told the true purpose of the study, and they did not give what we call today their "informed consent" when they agreed to be study subjects. The almost four hundred men in the study who had syphilis were not given adequate treatment for the disease or the choice to quit the study if they wanted to. When penicillin became available to treat syphilis in 1947, it was not offered to the men.

More recently, the case of Henrietta Lacks has fueled distrust of clinical research and healthcare systems as relates to Black people.[15] Lacks was a Black woman and mother of five who was treated at Johns Hopkins Hospital in 1951 for cervical cancer. While she was undergoing treatment, a sample of cells from her cervix was retrieved without her knowledge and sent to a nearby research lab that had been trying to grow tissues in culture. The researcher observed that Lacks's cells could be kept alive and grew indefinitely; these were the first "immortal" human cells ever grown in culture.

After Lacks died at age thirty-one, these "HeLa" cells (named for her first and last name) were used in numerous medical experiments and contributed to dozens of medical breakthroughs—including the development of the polio vaccine, in vitro fertilization, cloning, and gene mapping—and the study of HIV/AIDS and cancer treatments. The HeLa cells have been used in approximately half of the research that led to Nobel Prizes in medicine over the past sixty years. These cells have been an extraordinary gift to society.

Twenty-five years after Lacks died, some of her family members became involved in the research again without fully understanding what they were doing or what their biospecimens would be used for. Eventually, family members discovered that Lacks's cells had been commercialized, and even though the medical researchers who patented her tissue were making millions of dollars in profit, the family was not benefiting at all. Cases like these where Black people have been misled or not completely informed contribute to the running narrative that healthcare systems operated primarily by white people cannot be trusted.

I turn now to a story of one of my first mentors, that is a prime example of a strong Black woman who dedicated her life to caring for her community while enduring social stressors and trying to live up to the cultural expectation of the strong Black woman—at the ultimate sacrifice of her own mental health.

By my sophomore year at Cornell University, after struggling with depression and anxiety in high school and having my requests for therapy rebuffed by my parents, I declared my major in psychology. Over winter break and the following summer, I got my first psychology-related job working for a woman I'll call Dr. Kenyatta Jackson, the only clinical psychologist I knew, who also happened to be Black. I worked for Dr. Jackson at the mental health and substance abuse treatment center that she had founded, Jackson Integrated Healthcare.

Through her center, Dr. Jackson employed psychiatrists, psychologists, and mental health workers who provided individual, group, and family counseling and case management. The center included a twenty-bed substance abuse residential program where patients lived onsite and were treated for drug and alcohol addictions. I spent most of my time following her around to various community events, organizing her extensive home library, and calling to verify contact and disability claims information for hundreds of people who had been seen in the residential program. I was in awe of the work that she was doing for her people.

Even her home clearly exhibited that she was a woman with a distinct worldview centered on all things related to Black culture and the Black lived human experience. Floor-to-ceiling bookcases were overstuffed with books; boxes in the middle of the floor overflowed with books; and African diaspora art was dispersed throughout her condo, all displaying the brilliance and chaos of her fast-moving mind.

This quintessential scholar seemed thrilled by the naive optimism and ingenuity of youth. When us twenty-somethings gathered together in her home, she would lightly insert her ideas of how we could convene and *party with a purpose*. She saw the power within us and eagerly encouraged us to use it to uplift our community.

Three years after my internship with Dr. Jackson, things rapidly started to unravel for her. According to Dr. Jackson, her billing provider erroneously, and without her knowledge, submitted thousands of dollars of claims under a psychiatrist's name who worked for her rather than under the business's name. The eventual upshot was that her clinical psychology license was revoked after she was convicted for vendor fraud and theft for billing Medicaid for more than $400,000 in psychiatric and substance abuse services that were either never provided or were provided by unlicensed counselors employed at Jackson Integrated Healthcare. Although she was charged criminally, some community members saw her acts as merely "Robin Hooding" the system in order to provide mental health and substance abuse treatment to the most disenfranchised. Her sentence included six months in prison.

After Dr. Jackson was released from prison and on parole, her mental health and functioning deteriorated quickly, and she was no longer able to work. She supported herself with the help of public assistance and family members, who were unable to distinguish between her increasingly delusional thoughts and the truth. She believed that she had been wrongfully convicted, adamantly claimed her innocence, and refused to abide by the terms of her release. After violating her parole, she fled to Washington, DC, to hide out with her brother. She believed that she was being persecuted, watched, and followed by federal law enforcement. According to her, the feds had first gone looking for her in Chicago and then showed up in DC, pounding at the door with guns.

When she returned to Chicago, Dr. Jackson spent months, which turned into years, at the University of Chicago Law School library conducting legal research and learning to file legal briefs so that she could appeal her case and redeem her professional reputation. But her initial interest in learning the law to overturn her conviction transitioned into compulsively filing lawsuits against various individuals and corporations that she believed had harmed her. She believed that she would win a multimillion-dollar lawsuit that would allow her to buy her four children luxurious homes. She made lofty plans to buy a neighborhood bank and squandered her children's inheritance in an attempt to actualize these plans. Eventually, she moved on to writing a script for a television show in which the political climate of the Trump administration was acted out through characters from the *Wizard of Oz*. When one set of plans fell through, she would quickly move on to the next, leaving the remnants of her impulsivity and destructive behavior behind.

Her family suspected that she might have a mental health issue, but they were wary of confronting her about it. Initially, they had been supportive, but eventually they tired of her irrational beliefs and lack of accountability and pleaded that she let go of the past and pull herself back together. They, like many people, didn't understand how her untreated mental health condition prevented her from being able to function the way that she had in the past.

Dr. Jackson was easily able to use her intellect to almost persuade those around her that she was "fine" and simply a victim of a series of bad circumstances. She was so smart and accomplished that people dismissed her erratic behavior. For years she had been able to hide her mental health condition behind her contributions to the community and her successful career. Surely, she was more aware than most people of the stigma and potential consequences associated with mental illness and treatment. An attempt to preserve her reputation might have partly dissuaded her from getting the help that she needed.

Dr. Jackson demonstrated symptoms consistent with bipolar disorder. During periods of mania, she would focus intensely on a project and be productive—such as investigating her legal case or writing television scripts. Her mind would move fast and be full of fresh ideas. She also would make risky and impulsive decisions, particularly pertaining to money and business ventures. She believed that she was uniquely talented and powerful (which arguably she was). Then, predictably, she would become depressed and retreat from the world until the thrill of euphoria returned. This skilled psychologist appeared to have no insight into her irrational thoughts and behavior and did not see a need for mental health treatment.

But her physician eventually referred her for such treatment. Dr. Jackson went to one therapy session but then minimized the necessity of continued treatment by stating that the doctor had made the recommendation only because she had "been through so much in the past few years" and not because something was actually out of balance.

Unfortunately, for the past decade Dr. Jackson's mental health has continued to decline. She lives in public housing for seniors and is frequently at risk of being evicted. She has withheld the rent and filed multiple lawsuits against the building manager, the building management company, and the Chicago Housing Authority, claiming that the apartment isn't being kept in livable condition and as a result she gets rashes on her skin and has difficulty breathing. *Do Not Enter* and *No Trespassing* signs are posted on the door to her apartment, as she believes that people have entered her home without her permission.

Dr. Jackson's current state is a reflection of years of an undiagnosed mental health condition, exacerbated by incarceration and a lack of mental health treatment. Black people represent about 40 percent of those who are incarcerated in the United States despite being only about 14 percent of the population.[16] Sixty-four percent of people in jail and 56 percent of people in state prisons have some kind of mental health condition, and 10 to 25 percent have a serious mental health condition, like bipolar disorder. Cook County Jail in Chicago has been called the largest mental health provider in the nation because of the large numbers of people with mental health problems who pass through it each year.

Imprisonment can create new or exacerbate old mental health problems. While in prison, people are no longer able to engage in productive activities, such as work, that they may have been involved in on the outside. They may withdraw and isolate themselves. Prison is also a dangerous place, so people who are imprisoned can become suspicious, distrusting, and hypervigilant for signs of threat. Over time, delusions and paranoia can worsen.

With regard to the recognition and acceptance of mental health issues in the Black community, the tide has recently been turning with celebrities like actress Taraji P. Henson and radio personality and actor Charlamagne Tha God speaking up about them. These conversations in public spaces with large audiences are critical to recognizing the commonality of mental health challenges, reducing the shame and stigma people with these challenges experience, and encouraging people to seek mental health treatment.

"Being strong" is not believing that you have to handle everything on your own; instead, being strong is recognizing when you need help and using the resources that are available to you to get help. In addition to in-person therapy, there is a new wave of online community support, education, and resources specifically for the mental health needs of Black women, including:

- Therapy for Black Girls, founded by clinical psychologist Dr. Joy Harden Bradford
- Sista Afya Community Mental Wellness, founded by clinical social worker Camesha Jones
- Melanin & Mental Health, founded by therapists Eliza Boquin and Eboni Harris
- Black Mental Wellness, founded by clinical psychologists Drs. Nicole Cammack, Danielle Busby, Dana Cunningham, and Jessica Henry
- Girl Trek founded by Morgan Dixon and Vanessa Garrison
- *The Homecoming* podcast with clinical psychologist, ordained minister, and sacred artist Dr. Thema Bryant-Davis
- *Get Loved Up* podcast with wellness coach Koya Webb

Taking control of our mental health as Black women empowers us to be able to more effectively fulfill our roles as providers, caretakers, and community leaders. We must take a moment to be still and breathe deeply so that we have the emotional and physical strength to be well enough to be in service to others.

ELEVEN

The Breakdown

Although we Black women show up with dignity, grace, and composure, many of us may be privately breaking down, overcome with sadness or worry, withdrawing and isolating from friends and family, staying in bed all day, unable to function, or even contemplating death. When these feelings build up and boil over, we can be riddled with shame and guilt and incorrectly assume that we're the only ones going through such things. We believe that strong Black women aren't allowed the convenience of a break or breakdown.

Even when we are suffering, we think that we should be able to handle our feelings on our own without family support (they might tell your business) or professional support (you can't trust white counselors). When "being strong" means not acknowledging one's true feelings or asking for help, "being strong" leads to breaking down and upholding the façade that precludes healing.

As we have seen, Amber experienced chronic instability in childhood due to having a mentally ill mother and grandmother, living in poverty, and the impacts of racism. She lost her father because of divorce, her mother because of incarceration and death, and even her brother because he committed suicide (more on this in the next chapter). Amber endured these traumatic experiences heroically, and she developed into a strong Black woman, but her emotional anguish lay just below the surface, waiting to boil over.

Even in extreme despair, Amber couldn't bring herself to get help. When she lost her job, she felt like she was at the lowest point that she had ever been in her life. Soon thereafter, she found a therapist and scheduled an appointment, but she never showed up. She was ashamed and embarrassed about not being able to keep her emotions under control. It had been ingrained in her that you couldn't talk about your feelings. She was taught that if people saw her vulnerabilities, they would ultimately use them against her.

We Black women tend to believe this because we have suffered so many deep betrayals and hurts throughout our lives. So we show people that we're strong all the time—that whatever you throw at us, we can handle it. "There's the you at home and the you out there in the world. No one is ever supposed to see the pain," Amber said.

Amber was able to grind through the difficult period after losing her job, but she worried about her long-term mental health. It was hard for her to even imagine a life where pain didn't prevail. Whenever the next bad thing happened, she didn't think she'd be able to control her feelings anymore.

I encouraged my friend to seek mental health treatment to help her cope with her current suffering and to prepare for the future life challenges that would inevitably come. I suggested that she ask her primary care physician for therapist referrals, suggested she search the *Psychology Today* database, and offered her some referrals of Black women psychologists in private practice. She was concerned that a therapist would judge her and not understand her. I explained that it might take time to find a therapist who felt like a good fit.

I let Amber know that it might be hard to talk about her past in therapy. Since people who have experienced trauma often avoid reminders of the trauma, including talking about it, therapy might not always feel good. But talking allows you the opportunity to acknowledge what you have been through, hold space for the painful feelings, and learn how to cope with these feelings so that you can move from suffering toward healing.

Amber continued to avoid seeking mental health treatment. But a few years later when she found out that she had to have uterine fibroids removed at only age thirty, she hit her next valley. For weeks she felt depressed and withdrew from friends, and this time she was unable to shake it off.

On Thanksgiving Day in 2019, she experienced yet another traumatic loss. Her close friend Chauntelle Bernard was murdered by her husband, Dudley Bernard, a Customs and Border Protection officer.[1] He shot Chauntelle multiple times while their two sons were in the home. Amber was aware that Chauntelle had been experiencing domestic abuse, had seen videos of Dudley threatening her with weapons, and even had accompanied Chauntelle to get a restraining order. However, whenever Chauntelle tried to get help, she felt the authorities made it difficult and protected Dudley because he was a law enforcement officer.

Amber sank into a deeper depression after her friend's death. She cried all day while at work and at home, and for the first time, she started drinking excessively. She drank two to three bottles of wine every day in order to feel numb and distract herself from painful thoughts while she was awake and to help her fall asleep at night. Her mind constantly replayed all of the events leading up to Chauntelle's death. Guilt crept in, and she wondered whether she should have done more to help her. Painful thoughts about her mother and brother also began to resurface. Amber felt herself slipping and didn't think she could get out of it on her own. She was approaching rock bottom.

Amber finally decided that her symptoms were so severe that she needed to talk to someone. She knew that she didn't want medication, as she didn't think it was *that serious*. She asked her primary care physician to recommend a therapist, preferably a Black woman. She made an appointment—and rescheduled it twice. It was challenging for her to accept that she needed help. Talking to a therapist about her feelings and difficulty functioning would be a major step outside of the norm that had been established in her family. She didn't want anyone to have the misconception that something was wrong with her, although she felt weak and ashamed.

Amber finally showed up to her first therapy session, feeling nervous and overwhelmed. But the therapist truly seemed to want to get to know her, which made her feel more comfortable. She found the therapist to be a good listener, empathetic, and not judgmental. Her fears started to wane.

Amber had a lot of issues in her life—she had acute symptoms of depression, anxiety, and panic and had suffered multiple traumas. Even though therapy could not change past difficult life experiences, Amber appreciated having a safe space to be able to learn new and healthy ways to cope with her emotions.

Therapy helped her to reestablish her day-to-day routine, which had fallen by the wayside. Amber started to understand the weight of the trauma that she had been carrying and that had been made heavier by the pressure and expectation to "be strong." She released the shame and guilt that she had been clinging to. She started looking for places in her life where she could be just a little bit easier on herself and offer herself grace. If nothing else, therapy normalized her feelings and helped her realize that her feelings were not crazy. She found therapy to be empowering, and it felt good to know that she was doing something proactive to take care of herself.

Many Black women don't perceive a pressing need for treatment. Even if they do identify a problem, they believe that they can solve it on their own, that it will eventually get better with time, or that mental health treatment won't do any good. *A therapist can't change my situation*, they tell themselves. But in fact, a therapist can give *you* the tools to help *you* change your situation. For some, talking to a therapist is no different than talking to a friend or pastor.

In general, Black adults tend to have more negative attitudes and stigmatizing beliefs about mental illness and treatment, such as shame and self-blame, and they believe that others are not sympathetic toward people with mental health challenges.[2] Even Black women who are highly educated, successful, and have access to resources can have trouble climbing the hurdle of stigma to seek mental health treatment.

Dr. Jackson had been a prominent and well-respected expert in mental illness and substance abuse prevention and treatment, child welfare, and corrections throughout Chicago and nationwide. She graduated at the top of her college class and went on to earn graduate degrees in clinical psychology from a top-ranked university; she was the only Black student in her doctoral program. In 1975, she became one of the first Black women to be licensed as a psychologist in Illinois. She was an influential leader in professional organizations and a mentor for Black psychologists and other mental health professionals across the country. However, Dr. Jackson was never able to seek out and receive the help that she worked so hard to provide to others.

When I am working with women in therapy, they often do not lead with their trauma, but we gradually approach it as we begin a guided exploration into the situations that have led to their present distress. Beneath the surface problem is a set of life experiences, embedded within a family system and combined with individual biology and the social environment. In therapy we work to understand how all of these factors have contributed to the current state of suffering and replace learned unhealthy behaviors with new ones that promote wellness.

My client Heaven and I worked together in therapy to understand the root of her physical and emotional pain—her history of childhood sexual abuse—and the current situations that were triggering her depression and anxiety symptoms: her pending hysterectomy, the fear that she would not be able to have more children, and her feeling like a failure as a wife, mother, and woman. Therapy helped her to realize the connection between her physical body and emotional state and how much her physical pain, and the retraumatization it caused, triggered her depression, anxiety, and panic.

In therapy I help people to understand that thoughts such as "I'm worthless" and "Nobody loves me" and "I deserve for bad things to happen to me" are not facts, but rather mental events that we create in our minds. I worked with Heaven to disentangle her distorted, emotionally laden thoughts from her rational, reasonable mind and to help her to see her inherent, unconditional self-worth.

But Heaven resisted a more balanced, positive view of herself and instead firmly believed the negative thoughts in her mind to be true. She had been telling herself that she was no good for so long that she had a hard time seeing things any other way. She believed that the narrative that she had created about her worthlessness was fact. The hand of trauma that she was continuously dealt was evidence that the negative thoughts she had about herself *must* be true. She had a hard time seeing things any other way.

Heaven and I also worked together to identify the situations that triggered her fear, worry, and panic, which could occur almost anytime and anywhere. She felt anxious at work, walking around in her high-crime neighborhood, during intimacy with her husband, and whenever her daughter was not at home. She felt safe in very few places. Nonetheless, we designated a few areas—the broom closet at work and her bedroom at home—where she could go and calm herself when she felt anxious or panicky.

Heaven felt very alone and did not trust many people. We worked to identify two people—her sister and husband—she could share her feelings with and turn to for support. Heaven could rationally state that her husband was loving, supportive, and loyal, but she nonetheless was reluctant to be vulnerable and talk to him about her anxiety and depression.

It was difficult for Heaven to confront her trauma. I could feel the palpable tension between her wanting to talk about past painful situations and the present pain that she experienced when bringing these situations to mind. She clung to the ideals of the strong Black woman and felt that she was "less than" because she could not meet this standard.

After four sessions, Heaven started no-showing for appointments. When I called her, she said that she was so depressed that she couldn't leave her home. I reminded her that it is during these times that the safe space of therapy can be most important. The last time that I saw her, she was still in a lot of distress.

As a result of my client Gloria's genetic predisposition to traumatic stress and the trauma environment where she directly experienced childhood sexual abuse and intimate partner violence, she suffered from a number of mental and physical health conditions. She had a history of morbid obesity, a rare and painful inflammation of the layer of fat under the skin, and high cholesterol. About six months before starting therapy, she had gastric bypass surgery and was down to 170 pounds from more than 300 pounds. She had changed to a vegan diet and ate only small portions. She was proud of the weight that she'd lost, although people at her church told her that she was "too skinny" and looked "sick," which caused her to doubt the steps that she was taking to heal.

For years Gloria had used food and work as escape-avoidance strategies to cope with her post-traumatic stress. She worked twelve- to fourteen-hour days to avoid being at home, alone, in her studio apartment. Then one day, she passed out at work and had to be carried out by the paramedics. When she could no longer use work to avoid her thoughts and feelings, she became even more depressed. At night, when she felt lonely and sad, she ate butter cookies. "Sweets are my happy place," she told me. Within the first two years after her gastric bypass surgery, she gained back eighty of the pounds that she had lost.

Emotionally, Gloria at times felt numb or despondent and other times keyed up, anxious, and panicky. She had low self-esteem and judged herself harshly, not believing that she was as smart or as beautiful as other people. She had difficulty falling and staying sleep. Most nights she slept for only three to four hours. She avoided falling into deep sleep because she feared she would be vulnerable to someone coming into her apartment to harm her. The lack of sleep made her feel even more down, irritable, and on edge.

Gloria and I worked together in weekly therapy for more than five years. In the beginning, therapy provided her with a model relationship of trust, mutual respect, and boundaries. She learned that there could be a consistent and caring person in her life who would listen and provide honest feedback and coping skills with compassion and without judgment. With that foundation, we worked to identify and challenge the negative thoughts that she had about herself and her fear of abandonment and rejection. I reflected to Gloria that her thoughts were often stuck ruminating about past traumatic events, which led to invasive feelings of guilt and self-blame in the present. I helped her to see that the negative thoughts that she had about herself were the messages that she had internalized from the abuse from her father and ex-husbands.

Gloria and I reconstructed the view that she had of herself. She noticed when she was personalizing and taking the blame for the bad behavior of others, reading people's minds and assuming that they saw her as negatively as she saw herself, and discounting when she received positive affirmation from loved ones and overexaggerating what she perceived to be negative interactions.

Gloria identified her strengths as being kind, giving, thoughtful, and encouraging. She even started to feel good about her appearance, taking pride in her smooth skin, hairstyles, and fashion sensibility. As she became more sure of herself, she feared rejection less and was able to establish and maintain healthy relationships with others. By dealing with her trauma, Gloria was able to dig out of the hurt and to create a space for healing.

I encouraged Gloria to consider the behavioral steps that she could take in the present moment that would increase her opportunities for joy. For example, she loved being with people and identified those who loved her to whom she could reach out to talk to or spend time with. She also enjoyed many hobbies, such as finding new recipes, experimenting with her hair, rearranging her apartment, and going to the movies or thrift stores, and she made time to do these things.

These behavioral strategies kept Gloria in the present moment rather than in the suffering of her traumatic past. As her mood started to improve, she enrolled in an associate's program and volunteered in hospice care. After she completed her degree, she began working as a caregiver, where she could use her love of people in service to others, especially the elderly. Gloria thrived in this space and called her caregiving clients her "friends." Now back at work, she had a sense of purpose and felt productive and valued. Her sense of self-worth improved dramatically. She had less time to focus on the negative thoughts that had previously preoccupied her. She constantly received praise from her supervisors and her "friends" and always gave the glory to God.

Now that her depression had waned, she was ready to tackle the weight that she had gained back. She started a structured meal plan and stuck to it consistently. Rather than feel restricted, she felt good that she was doing something to take control of her life. As someone who loved to cook and try new things, she relished making healthy and tasty recipes. In nine months Gloria lost those eighty pounds—in a healthy way. She said that she was living her "best life." These days, she holds her head up high and smiles.

TWELVE

Black People Don't Commit Suicide

There is a dangerous false narrative that Black people don't kill themselves. However, a history of trauma, which Black women are vulnerable to, as we have seen, is a key risk factor for suicide. In 2018 in the United States, suicide was one of the top four leading causes of death among individuals aged ten to fifty-four and the tenth leading cause of death overall.[1] According to the Centers for Disease Control and Prevention, in 2019 a person died by suicide every eleven minutes.[2]

The most common factor contributing to death by suicide, nearly half the time, is a relationship problem. Other issues include an upcoming crisis (29 percent), excessive substance use (28 percent), a physical health problem (22 percent), a job/financial problem (16 percent), or a criminal/legal problem (9 percent).[3] Some of the reasons that my clients tell me they have considered suicide include a recent loss of a relationship, feeling stuck in a violent relationship, financial problems causing them to face homelessness, feeling alone or abandoned by family, and feeling as if nobody would care or miss them if they were gone.

Although men are more likely than women to complete a suicide, women are more likely than men to attempt one. White people are three times as likely to commit suicide than Black and Hispanic people (15.8 percent, 5.6 percent, and 5.8 percent, respectively).[4] Out of white men, white women, Black men, and Black women, Black women are least likely to commit suicide. The apparent lack of suicidal behavior among Black women compared with white and nonwhite men has been called "the black-white suicide paradox."

However, suicide is not unheard of in the Black community. The rate of suicide attempts and deaths by suicide among Black people has been increasing for the past twenty years. Among Black women, the suicide rate increased by a staggering 65 percent from 1999 to 2017.[5] Astonishing increases have also been seen among Black youth. From 1991 to 2017, rates of suicide attempts for Black youth increased by 73 percent.[6] From 2001 to 2017, rates of suicide for Black boys ages thirteen to nineteen increased by 60 percent and rates for Black girls increased by 182 percent.[7]

These increases are partly due to the stress that can come from living in the United States as a Black person. The 2018 suicide of nine-year-old McKenzie Adams of Linden, Alabama, is a tragic example of a Black youth who experienced stress in the form of bullying at school. It is also a chilling example of how children's social environments can have a fatal impact on their mental and emotional functioning if adequate protections aren't in place to recognize when they are vulnerable and to intervene appropriately. McKenzie's mother said that in the months leading up to her death, her daughter endured persistent racist bullying at school. She rode to school every day with a white family friend and was taunted with words such as "You think you're white because you ride with that white boy," "Black bitch," "you're ugly," "kill yourself," and "just die."

Although her mother said that McKenzie told her teachers and the assistant principal that she was being harassed, the school denies any knowledge of the bullying. According to the Centers for Disease Control and Prevention, youth who report high levels of bullying are more likely to report high levels of suicide-related behavior than those who do not experience bullying behavior.[8]

Despite such increasing suicide rates among Blacks, there is a sweeping lack of awareness about the presence of suicidal thoughts, suicide attempts, and death by suicide in the Black community. Often, Black people at high risk for suicide are silent about their thoughts and plans to commit suicide and so are not helped or treated. This information gap is maintained by the notion of infallible resilience and all-enduring strength that denies our vulnerability to suicide and fuels secrecy when a suicide does occur.

When actress Halle Berry admitted that she had attempted suicide after her divorce from baseball player David Justice, she was not spared any criticism or offered compassion. Instead, the public discourse asserted that if someone as rich and beautiful as Berry had considered suicide, she *must* be crazy.

Firearms are the most common method of suicide among Black men and women, followed by hanging.[9] More than among any other demographic group, suicides among Black people are more likely to be misclassified as being due to other causes of death. For example, when a death involving prescription pills, illicit drugs, or alcohol is reported, it can be unclear whether it was a suicide or an accident, as in the case of singer Whitney Houston in 2012. Additionally, when deaths involve police, such as in the 2015 case of Sandra Bland, who was found hanged in her jail cell, it can be unclear whether the death was a suicide or a murder.

Halle Berry stopped the attempt to take her own life when she became fearful of what the afterlife would be like for someone who committed suicide. Acknowledging thoughts of suicide for some people would mean that they had lost faith in God—one of the deadliest of sins in the Black community. Scripture teaches Christians, "Trust in the Lord with all your heart, / and do not lean on your own insight. / In all your ways acknowledge him, / and he will make straight your paths" (Prov 3:5–6, NRSV). Have faith that things will get better, we are told. Do not take things into your own hands. Scripture also promises punishment if one harms oneself: "Do you know that you are God's temple and that God's Spirit dwells in you? If anyone destroys God's temple, God will destroy that person. For God's temple is holy, and you are that temple" (1 Cor 3:16–17, NRSV).

While religious practices and spiritual beliefs are an effective coping strategy for many, those who cannot overcome their painful emotions in spite of their faith may keep their suicidal thoughts to themselves in fear of ridicule and shame.

Black women's commitment to religious beliefs can be protective against suicide. Research has found that African Americans who attend religious services at least once a week and say that they "look to God for strength" are less likely to attempt suicide.[10] Similarly, women who attend religious services once a week or more have five times lower risk for committing suicide.[11] Participation in religious activities embeds people in a network of social support and protects them against the loneliness and isolation that can come with depression. People who are contemplating suicide are often bogged down by hopelessness, and religion can provide hope and the belief that their suffering has a purpose. Religion provides a safety net.

In addition to religion, familial support and being embedded in a kinship network are important protective factors for suicide, especially among Black women. The idea of leaving our children or other loved ones to fend for themselves is unconscionable. We feel a selfless devotion to others and believe we have to show up for those whom we love. We don't want to disappoint or let anyone down.

On the other hand, people such as the women we have met in these pages who have suffered sexual, physical, and emotional abuse at the hands of family members may fall into a deep depression and have suicidal thoughts when it seems that the despair just won't let up. And if they have few meaningful connections to family, friends, work, and community that can help them feel productive and valued, they can be particularly vulnerable to suicide.

The trauma that my friend Amber endured, combined with the pressure and expectation that she put on herself to compensate for her mother's mental illness, contributed to her depression as an adolescent. She had days when she didn't want to get up or do anything. On some nights she played with her mom's kitchen knife sets, contemplating death. Eventually, she felt so hopeless that she attempted suicide, taking as many of the pills as she could find in the medicine cabinet. Luckily, her mother found her and took her to the hospital. But the suicide attempt triggered an investigation of Amber's mother for neglect. She feared social services prying into what was happening in the household and taking her children away. The case, however, was ultimately deemed unfounded.

Four months after Amber's mother died, her younger brother committed suicide by jumping into the Chicago River and drowning. Since that day, feelings of guilt and self-blame for her brother's death have haunted Amber. She wonders whether she should have been more upfront with him about their mother's illness rather than trying to protect him by withholding information.

Amber's family refused to talk about the suicide, preferring to deny, through silence, the truth of what happened. To them, suicide was something Black people just didn't do. While there is certainly stigma attached to mental illness, the stigma associated with suicide is even more deep-seated, especially in religious southern Black families. We tend to think that by not disclosing information we are protecting loved ones from pain and suffering, but we may be leaving room for them to fill in the gaps of the unknown with distorted explanations. By having difficult conversations, we create space to share fears and information, seek mutual understanding, and dispel the power of the unknown.

Amber managed to turn the difficult circumstance of suicide in her family into awareness. On her brother's birthday she honors his life and speaks up about suicide on social media. In one post she wrote to her brother: "Suicide ripped you from the world and you were still just a boy. I wish I could've done more, felt more, understood more. I wish your casket could've been opened so I could say goodbye and hug you one more time. Happy birthday baby brother. Give Mom a hug for me."

Like Amber, I also had thoughts of suicide when I was an adolescent. The summer after eighth grade, depression had really set in. Combined with everything that was going on at home, I felt awkward and as if I didn't fit in at school. I was upset with my mom, who wouldn't leave the situation with my father, as he pinged back and forth between two families.

One Saturday afternoon, I found myself sitting in my bedroom with the window cracked open, listening to the sounds of voices buzzing below me, thinking about death. I thought, *Maybe if I was gone, that would get my parents' attention and they'd realize how much they're hurting me.* Then the familiar retort, *Nobody is hurting you; you're fine*, played over in my mind, but I couldn't reconcile it with the agony that I felt in the moment.

I nervously scrambled through the bathroom cabinet, found a bottle of Tylenol, took about ten pills, and waited with anticipation for something to happen. About twenty minutes later I started feeling a little drowsy and heard my cousin calling my name from the bottom of the steps. The stairs creaked as he walked up to my room and then sat on the bed next to me. "What's wrong?" he asked. I told him that I wasn't feeling well and had taken some Tylenol. "You'll be okay; you're fine," he said. I put my head down in his lap and cried as he silently rubbed my back.

In a mindfulness group I conducted a few years ago for Black women with depression, one young woman in her early twenties declared outright, "Sometimes I get so depressed I think about killing myself." She held nothing back and had moved past caring what other people thought about her. "I just can't take this bullshit no more," she continued. She was frustrated and tired. Dying seemed like the only way to escape the all-encompassing depression she felt.

She had a two-year-old and a three-year-old and was seven months pregnant. A recent study found that in the year before and after giving birth, suicidal thoughts and self-harm nearly tripled among childbearing people.[12] This woman's pregnancy was considered high risk, so she was on bed rest and could no longer work. She had experienced postpartum depression after her last pregnancy, and now she was depressed again. Her boyfriend spent most of his time hustling in the streets, and the two of them were into it all the time.

She held up both of her wrists to reveal the dark scars showing where she had cut herself before with a butcher knife to release the pain. The room fell silent. Some of the women stared at her with wretched concern, and others looked away.

After the session was over, I approached her. She seemed impatient and annoyed that I wanted to talk more; she rolled her eyes and turned her shoulders away. But she didn't walk away. Before long, she unwound and the irritation melted away. She said that she thought about suicide all the time, mostly because "I don't have nobody."

She realized the tension in her relationship was not good for the baby she was carrying. But she was stuck in the house all day and couldn't go out and do anything. Sometimes she wished that she had never had her kids. She didn't know how she was going to take care of them and didn't have any support. Her mom and sisters were always in her business and talked about her behind her back.

When I asked her whether she experienced any abuse in her relationship, her eyes cut upwards, then off to the side. "Nah," she said. I asked her whether she'd had any plans for how she might harm herself and whether she had any intention to do so in the future. She said that she didn't have any plans, but sometimes she thought that everything would be easier if she were dead. I assessed her access to lethal items such as knives, pills, and guns and created a safety plan to eliminate or minimize her exposure to these items. She agreed that she would call her primary care doctor if the suicidal thoughts became more persistent and she could not control them, and she would go to the emergency room if she was in a state of immediate crisis. We talked about how she might get connected to therapy. When I followed up with her the next day, she didn't answer, and I never heard from her again. Far too often, women like this are not identified as being high-risk for suicide and fall through the cracks of the system.

The loss of a loved one who has completed a suicide can be complex and traumatic. Death by suicide is usually sudden and unexpected and sometimes violent, which contributes to its traumatic effects. Family members grapple with intense mixed emotions, ranging from abandonment to guilt, and even anger. They ask themselves "what if" and question whether they could have done something to prevent the death. However, survivors tend to greatly overestimate their contributing role in the death and the role they believe they could have played in its prevention.

People who have lost someone to suicide are at increased risk for having thoughts of suicide themselves and making an attempt. People often contemplate death because they want to relieve insufferable pain or because they feel hopeless and don't see things getting better in the future. But even in the darkest moments of suffering, there is light ahead if we reach for it and accept its invitation to move forward.

If you find yourself having thoughts of suicide, know that while you might feel overwhelmed and hopeless in the moment, the intensity of emotions rises and falls, like the tide of an ocean's wave. Resist the urge to take a permanent action to address a temporary feeling. Identify things in your life that give you hope and purpose—like people you love and who love you. If you are having trouble identifying something, know that you are valuable just because you are a living, breathing human being. You don't have to *do* anything or prove anything to be worthy of living and love.

Reach out to someone and let them know how you are feeling and the thoughts that you are having—perhaps a friend or a pastor or even your primary care doctor. You can also call the National Suicide Prevention Lifeline, available for free, twenty-four hours a day, seven days a week, at 800-273-8255. Get rid of things that you could use to impulsively cause yourself harm, like unnecessary medications or weapons.

Finally, when you have come out of the eye of the storm, create a hope box and include in it a letter to remind yourself of what you've been through and, most importantly, that you overcame. Tell yourself how you did it so that should you ever feel this way again, you can come back to the letter. You may also include other things in the box that give you joy, like pictures of loved ones, mementos from special places you've been, or reminders of things you'd like to do or places you'd like to go in the future. Open up this box from time to time and be reminded of the things that have brought you joy in the past and what you look forward to in the future.

HEALING

Heartbreak opens onto the sunrise
For even breaking is opening
And I am broken
I'm open
Broken to the new light without pushing in
Open to the possibilities within, pushing out
See the love shine in through my cracks?
See the light shine out through me?
I am broken
I am open
I am broken open
See the love light shining through me
Shining through my cracks
Through the gaps
My spirit takes journey
My spirit takes flight
Could not have risen otherwise
And I am not running
I'm choosing
Running is not a choice from the breaking
Breaking is freeing
Broken is freedom
I am not broken
I'm free.

DEE REES, from the movie *Pariah*

THIRTEEN

Maybe I Should Talk to Someone

People who have never been to therapy before are usually unsure of what to expect. They may conjure up the old Freudian image of a person lying supine on a dark leather couch with their eyes gazing up at the ceiling in a dimly lit room while a bearded male therapist sits behind them sterilely analyzing the words that fall out of their consciousness. Or they may think of the scene from the movie *One Flew over the Cuckoo's Nest* where a handcuffed Jack Nicholson is connected to electrodes and held down on a hospital bed as he violently convulses before an intimidating team of doctors and nurses dressed in white.

Regardless of the image that comes to mind, the underlying sentiment is often fear. *What is the therapist going to do to me? Are they going to be able to read my mind? Are they going to force me to talk about things I don't want to talk about? What are they going to do with the information? Are they going to judge me? Can talking to someone really make me feel better?* The thought of exposing the most vulnerable parts of yourself to a stranger can be terrifying. In the midst of myriad other responsibilities that Black women face daily, therapy can feel like one more thing that we just don't have time for.

When I meet clients for the first time, I explain to them that the first session or two will focus on collecting information about the problem that is bringing them to see me at that moment. Additionally, I ask questions about their early childhood development, school, work, social functioning, family history, history of physical and mental illnesses, and general medical and mental health treatment history. Finally, I query current signs, symptoms, and behavior patterns in order to make a preliminary diagnosis, if there is one. At the end of the session, clients and I discuss their goals for therapy and develop a treatment plan. Let me show you what a typical first therapy session might look like.

Brandy showed up for her ninety-minute intake appointment wearing her work badge. She was a social worker at a nearby hospital and squeezed the appointment in during her lunch break. When I came out to the waiting room to introduce myself, her eyes lit up and she smiled brightly.

We settled into my private office. She sat on the loveseat, and I sat in the armchair across from her. Notes from the previous session remained on the white board— *Mindfulness is paying attention, on purpose, in the present moment, without judgment.*

I started the session as I always do with new clients, by describing how today's session and future sessions would go. "Today, I'll take some time to get to know what brings you in, and I'd like to know a bit about your background. We'll end by developing a plan for how we'll go forward, and you'll have an opportunity to ask me questions. After our session, I'll make a note in your medical chart that will include a basic overview of what we've discussed. The things that you say in here are confidential, with some limits. If you express an intention to harm yourself or someone else, I have to take the necessary steps to keep you or that other person safe. If I learn of child or elder abuse, I also have a duty to report that. Outside of that, I'll always get your signed permission before speaking with anyone else. Is it okay for us to get started?"

Brandy nodded and then told me why she had sought out therapy. Her voice quavered and her eyes reddened as she spoke.

"About six months ago my sister's husband murdered her and then himself, and I've been having a hard time getting over it. Every time I drive past their house, which is every day, I get upset and start crying. I can't stop thinking about it. I find myself imagining how everything must've played out and wonder if I was driving down the block when he was killing her. They said he stabbed her six times, and there was a lot of blood."

I assured Brandy that most people who had gone through something like that would have a difficult time. I asked her whether she was having nightmares or flashbacks.

"I don't think so. I just get so upset and angry. Every time I see someone who looks like her husband, I get angry. How could he do that to her? Then I start looking at my boyfriend sideways, wondering if he might do something like that to me. I mean, I don't think he would, but I wonder." Her fingers curled in, as if she were squeezing the anger in her hands.

I asked her to tell me about her boyfriend. She smiled shyly and said they've been together four years, they live together, and they have a three-year-old son. "He's a good guy," she said. "He's amazing."

"How would you describe him?" I asked.

"He's very sweet, affectionate. He really loves our son, always teaching him things and playing with him. He's patient, hard-working. A really nice guy."

"That's good to hear. Sounds like he's an important source of support for you," I said. Brandy scooted back on the couch to get a bit more comfortable.

Then I said, "Let's return to the loss of your sister, if that's okay."

"Sure."

"You said that you get pretty upset, even angry, when you think about what happened to her. Do you find yourself avoiding reminders of her?"

"No, not really. I mean, I can't. She lived around the corner from my grandmother, and my grandmother babysits my son, so I drive past that block every day. Sometimes when I drive by it seems like I'm looking for her to be on the porch like she usually would be. Watering her flowers or something."

"Have you been inside of the house?"

"I went in once right after it happened, but I stayed downstairs. I couldn't bring myself to go upstairs where it happened." She looked up into her thoughts.

"Would you say you've felt down, depressed, or hopeless?" I asked.

"Not really, just sad."

"What about having little interest or pleasure in doing things? Do you feel like you don't want to be bothered with anything?"

Brandy thought for a moment. "No, I don't think I've felt that way."

"Do you find yourself worrying a lot and not being able to control it?"

"Yeah, I worry," she said. "Mostly about my son being safe. Also my grandmother. She's getting older and doesn't take care of herself. I worry about her health. My mom, she's still on and off the streets, so I worry about her too. Every day I have so much to do. I worry about keeping up and getting everything done." Brandy took in a deep breath and then released it.

"Do you ever find yourself feeling nervous, anxious, or on edge?" I asked.

"Yeah, my nerves are bad. There's so much going on out there, you just never know. I never know when the next bad thing is going to happen. My boyfriend says that I'm always worked up and get startled easy. Always jumping and what not." Brandy rolled her eyes and smiled coyly.

"Does that nervousness show up in your body? Like tightness in your neck or your stomach knotting up? Headaches? Shortness of breath?"

"My neck is always tensed up," she said. "Sometimes I clench my hands and don't even realize it."

"Are you ever able to relax?"

"Ain't never any time to relax. I'm always on the go."

I asked her about her sleep. "I don't get that much sleep," she said, "because I'm working, in school, and I have to take care of my son, but I sleep okay. By the end of the day I'm so tired, I fall out."

And her appetite? "It's fine, I've gained twenty pounds in the last few months, but I figure that's just stress. I been so busy with school." She looked up at me, shaking her head and pursing her lips, as if to say, *It is what it is.*

I asked about her physical health. "I have high blood pressure, but I guess that's just stress too. I'm trying to watch what I eat. I get migraines too."

Brandy told me that she had still been able to function—to make it to work and school without any trouble. "I get everything done," she said. "I don't really have a choice with that. I mean, if I don't do it, then who will?" Her eyebrows raised to question me.

"Do you ever find it difficult to concentrate or pay attention?" I asked.

"Sometimes my mind floats off, but it's not too bad. Mostly, I think about my sister, wondering if I missed something, what I could have done to help her. There was no violence in the relationship, far as we knew, but her husband had been addicted to heroin. They said he called his therapist three times that day and couldn't get in touch with him. He called the police and told them he was gonna do it, but they didn't get there in time. You know, they be slow getting to the neighborhood." I noticed that she was replaying the events, still trying to put the pieces together.

Brandy spoke softly and deliberately as I asked her questions. She sat upright on the loveseat and was calm and composed. When she spoke about her sister, her eyes teared up, and her gaze drifted out the window, as if she could see her.

Then I explored Brandy's background. She was from the West Side of Chicago. "My grandmother raised me and my sister because my mother was on drugs. My mother lived with us, but she was in and out. My dad was on drugs too, but he was around. He'd come and get us on the week-ends. We always loved going with him." She smiled fondly while remembering her dad.

"How would you describe your childhood?" I asked.

"It was good. I had everything I needed and didn't want for anything. It was always me and my sister. My cousins lived in the neighborhood too so it was fun to have them around. We did everything together."

I asked about middle school and high school. "I was a good student," she said, "into everything—cheerleading, dance troop, student council. I was homecoming queen all four years. Oh, and I worked part time at Nike. I loved always having nice clothes and the latest shoes. Still do." Brandy sat up a little straighter and ran her hand over her head to smooth her hair down.

"Sounds like you were pretty popular," I commented.

Trying to be modest, she answered, "Yeah, I had a lot of friends."

Brandy said she never had any trouble or problems at school, and when I asked whether she had experienced emotional, physical, or sexual abuse when she was a child, she answered: "No, not really. I mean, my mom could be kinda mean when she was in one of her moods, yelling and cussing at us and what not, but that's about it."

"What did you do after high school?"

"I went to college in Georgia. I did it all on my own. No one else in my family had been to college. My grandma supported me, but she couldn't do much to help financially. My dad was supposed to carry me down there, but on the day we were supposed to go, he never showed up. My auntie said he was off somewhere using. I had to get a bus ticket and get down there by myself. Just me and my lil' suitcase on the bus. I didn't talk to him for a while after that, but we're okay now." Sadness passed through quickly, and she pushed it away with a shrug—*Whatever.*

"How did you do in college?" I asked.

Modest pride returned as she answered: "I was an A student. I've always been real focused and determined. I worked while I was in school doing hair. I was always working and saving my money so I could have the things that I wanted. I even bought my own car."

"Sounds like you've always been pretty busy and productive."

"Yeah, I like it that way. You know, being independent. I've always had a lot of things going on and been able to take care of myself."

Then we moved on to what she was doing now, after college.

"I'm a social worker," she told me. "I like helping people. For the last two years I've been in school again, getting my doctorate so I can move up to administration."

"That's wonderful! What an accomplishment!" I wanted Brandy to know that it *was* a wonderful accomplishment.

Then it was time to explore a little deeper: "So far

you've shared with me the tragic loss of your sister. Have
you had any other very stressful life events involving actual
or threatened death, serious injury, or sexual violence?"

"Yeah, my cousin, one of the ones I told you about, he
was murdered on the block five years go." She paused briefly
and met my eyes, as if to say, *I hadn't thought about that.*

"I'm so sorry to hear that."

"He had just come outside to help my grandmother
bring in the groceries, and he got shot. Apparently they
were lookin' for someone else, but they got him. They
called me while I was at work, and I came running."

"Does anything else come to mind?"

"I'm not sure if this counts, but I had a miscarriage a
year ago. I was five months pregnant with a baby girl." Her
eyes welled up, and this time a tear fell. Her gaze trailed
down, and she started fidgeting.

"It makes me pretty sad to think about. I'm getting
older, and I want more kids. Me and my boyfriend have
been trying, but I haven't been able to get pregnant again."

I then thanked Brandy for everything she had shared
with me, acknowledging how hard it is to talk about such
things. I asked her a few more questions and found out
that she drank alcohol socially, and not very often. She also
had never used illegal drugs, "because of my parents," she
said. And this was the first time she had ever been to see a
therapist.

"I'm glad that you're here," I told her, and she smiled.

"Me too."

I also asked about whether anyone else in her family
had mental health problems, like depression or anxiety.

"I'm not sure," she said. "My mom say she depressed. But I think it's just the drugs."

Had Brandy ever felt so down that she had thoughts about death or dying? She shook her head firmly with disdain. "No, God no. I couldn't because of my son."

Then I asked her who she could turn to for help and support.

"Hmph, it's really me helping everybody else all the time," she said. "I don't ask for help too much. But I guess I could say my boyfriend. And maybe my granny too."

Before wrapping up, I asked her, "Is there anything that you think is important for me to know in this first session that we haven't talked about yet?"

She thought about it and then said, "Yeah, when you were asking me about my boyfriend. He's a good man, but sometimes I have trouble opening up to him and trusting him. He says I don't ever let him help me with anything. He wants to get married, but I'm scared. Especially after what happened with my sister."

I thanked her for adding that information and then summed up and told Brandy what she could expect from me in the future. "Based on what you've told me today, it sounds like you're struggling with general anxiety and grief because of the traumatic loss of your sister. You mentioned worry related to the safety and well-being of your family, being able to get everything done, and fear about the next bad thing happening. You also mentioned being keyed up and having difficulty relaxing, not getting much sleep, and recent changes in your appetite. Together, all of this sounds like anxiety. The anxiety is worsened by the other significant traumatic losses that you have experienced in your life. This is something that we can work on together in therapy.

"Although I did a lot of question-asking today, in our future sessions, I'll ask you to take the lead to share with me what you feel is most important to talk about in each session. I'll work with you to point out unhealthy thoughts and patterns of behavior that are contributing to the anxiety, anger, and grief that you're experiencing in the moment. I'll also give you some practical skills for coping with those emotions. Sometimes I'll ask you to do pen-and-paper homework, and other times I might give you a mental homework assignment that we'll discuss the next week in therapy. If you find that you're not getting what you need in our sessions, please let me know so that we can adjust. Therapy is a process of working together, and I want to make sure that I'm doing my part to help you to feel better."

Brandy said that it all sounded good to her. Then I asked her what her key goals for future therapy sessions would be. "It sounds like working on the anxiety and grief is one," I said. "What would you say are the others?"

"I think I want to talk about the miscarriage and my relationship with my boyfriend," she said.

"Great, I'll make sure that we have space to discuss those things and anything else that comes up." I asked Brandy how she felt about this first therapy session.

"It felt really good," she said. "The time went by so quick. I was worried about coming in here because I didn't know what to expect. But it was good to talk and get these things out."

As I did with Brandy, at the end of sessions I always check in with clients and ask them how it went from their perspective. Many times they exhale a sigh of relief and say that it wasn't as bad as they expected. The anticipation of what I would be like as a therapist is over. Although talking about painful experiences can be uncomfortable, clients usually say that it felt good to get things off their chest. Usually, they seem hopeful about continuing the process of therapy and healing.

On the basis of the information that clients provide from week to week, I help them to understand how past experiences have shaped the lens through which they see the world in the present. The loss of Brandy's sister, and the related grief and anger that she was experiencing, is what initially brought her to therapy. However, early on we discovered that other factors were contributing to her current anxiety, such as being raised in a chaotic household environment, her trauma history, family stress, and the multiple provider, caregiver, and work responsibilities that she was trying to manage. Brandy liked to have a plan and be in control of most things in her life. When something happened that she could not control, like the miscarriage, she felt very uneasy.

Common goals for therapy are to improve self-esteem, feel less sad, stop worrying so much, deal with family or relationship issues, or find a sense of direction or purpose in life. Sometimes people say that they just need a safe space to talk to someone without being judged because their family and friends don't understand what they are going through. A person may know that something is wrong— they feel down, less energetic and more sluggish, like they don't want to do anything, empty, and like they are just going through the motions. They are unable to pinpoint when the feeling started, why, or how to fix it. Occasionally, a person seeks help at the urging of a family member, a spouse, or a parent who has noticed that they are not acting like themselves and taking care of their responsibilities as they typically would.

Clients have different needs and show varying readiness to confront their distress. It is the therapist's job to meet clients where they are and go at a pace that they can handle. People with chronic stress may need help identifying the situational factors contributing to their stress, like feeling overextended and undersupported. I work with clients to take the steps within their control to manage the thoughts, physical reactions, and behaviors that are contributing to their stress.

We start by looking at everything on their plate, and I ask, "Does everything need to be on this list right now?" Then we can determine which tasks can be taken off entirely, which responsibilities can be reduced, and where help can be enlisted. Some clients need permission to simply be still without having to *do* all of the time. Others need a nudge to get unstuck so that they can take care of the high-priority things that they have been avoiding as well as participate in the enjoyable activities that they have been denying themselves.

Clients and I work together to identify unhealthy patterns of behavior that are sustaining distress. I helped Brandy to see how her desire to control everything at work, with family, in her relationship, which was driven by her worry that something might go wrong, and perfectionism, made her even more stressed because it meant that she had to do everything herself and was stretched too thin.

Brandy started to notice how stress showed up in her body— the way her heart started racing and she got short of breath when she realized that she was going to have to stay late at work and miss dinner with her son. When the trigger hit, she practiced a mindfulness technique called *STOP*: Stop, Take a Breath, Observe, and Proceed. Wherever she was, she paused for a few moments and slowed her breath down before deciding how to proceed.

Over time, Brandy became aware of the thoughts that played in her mind and contributed to her stress: *I have to be the one who picks up the extra work or else it's not going to get done; I should be there for my family because I'm the one who's made it; I have to do all the chores at home because my boyfriend isn't going to do it right.*

Strong Black women often take on too much responsibility and as a result are weighed down and burned out. We slip into believing that we should be able to be everything to everybody. It can feel like we don't have any choice other than to try and meet the unreasonable expectations of others, but we do. Choosing not to accept this passed-down burden does not make us less-than. In therapy, we challenge the triad of negative cognition: having negative thoughts about oneself (*I'm selfish if I don't help out all the time*), having negative thoughts about the future (*I'm going to have to take care of these people the rest of their lives*), and having negative thoughts about the world (*the world is full of people who just take from you and never give anything back*).

When people become more aware of the thoughts that play in their mind and realize that these messages are just stories told from one perspective and not necessarily the truth, they are empowered to create a new, affirming tape in their minds, they feel stronger, and in turn are better positioned to change their behavior. For instance, someone may ask you to run them to the store, and the thought might immediately pop up: *If I don't do it, they'll think that I feel I'm too good to help them out.* But instead, you might say to yourself: *It's okay to say* No *and go get my hair done instead. I took them to the* store last week and gave them $50. It's not my fault if they're angry. In this way you give yourself the same empathy that you would offer to a friend.

Changing our thoughts, and the expectations that we have for ourselves, frees us to do things in different, healthier ways. We take care of ourselves by not being afraid to say *No* or *Not right now* or *Let me think about it and get back to you*. Ask yourself, *What can I say* No *to today that no longer serves me?* Often we are reluctant to say *No* and set boundaries because it feels too uncomfortable to be on the receiving end of someone's disappointment or anger. It's true, people may become upset when you recalibrate the system that has been serving them. But this is a critical step in establishing new expectations and priorities that serve your wellness. We have to let go of feelings of guilt that come with not being able to meet everyone's expectations all the time. It is not your responsibility to be always available to meet everyone's needs. You don't have to be everyone's savior.

When you don't assert yourself by saying *No*, over time you can lose your voice and ultimately your power. In not setting boundaries we are reinforcing a system that prioritizes the other person's needs over our own. Sometimes saying *Yes* to someone else means that you are saying *No* to yourself. Identify your own wants and needs and align your behaviors so that your needs are being met. Use your voice to advocate for yourself. This goes for little things that at the surface seem like they don't matter, such as telling a family member that you don't always want to be expected to pick up the check when you go out to eat. It means asking for what you need, like thirty minutes of quiet time when you first get home. Speaking up in this way will allow you to feel more empowered and seen.

Removing the clutter of responsibilities can help you to clarify your priorities. Brandy decided that finishing school, doing a good job at work, and spending time with her son were priorities. In order to have space for these things, she looked carefully for opportunities to step back from running errands for family members (especially when they could do those errands themselves) and allow her boyfriend to help out more around the house (even if it wouldn't be exactly the way that she wanted it done). I also made sure that Brandy included self-care time as a priority so that she could get her hair and nails done, which she enjoyed.

No matter where each person begins, everybody is looking to be freed from suffering. Therapy is the process of identifying the source of our suffering, either in the past or the present; becoming aware of how we cling to that which causes us pain; and learning how to let it go. Therapy is one way to offer ourselves the time and space to heal.

In addition to individual therapy, someone might pursue *group therapy*, which is when a group of six to twelve people meet together with one or two facilitators. Groups usually meet once or twice a week for one to two hours. Although some groups are ongoing, most run from six to twelve sessions. Group participants share their experiences, learn coping skills, and receive support from the other group members. Therapy groups are usually put together around specific topics, such as dealing with grief, postpartum depression, or learning and practicing mindfulness.

A few years ago, I began a clinical research study to explore whether mindfulness practices would help women who were stressed, depressed, and anxious. *Mindfulness* is defined as the act of paying attention in a particular way, on purpose, in the present moment, and nonjudgmentally rather than running on autopilot.[1] Mindfulness practices can include sitting meditation, body visualization, and gentle yoga. The groups were run out of a community health center on the South Side of Chicago, where 93 percent of the residents are Black, 37 percent of households are led by a single mother, the unemployment rate is 27 percent, and 40 percent of people live below the federal poverty line.

Given the mental health stigma within the Black community that precludes many Black women from identifying themselves as needing help, the groups were advertised as women's wellness groups, rather than as mental health treatment. The brochure listed common symptoms of depression, such as feeling stressed, overwhelmed, and irritable; having difficulty paying attention or concentrating; feeling tense or on edge; feeling unmotivated; having difficulty sleeping; and feeling fatigue. Women saw themselves in these symptoms, even when they adamantly denied being depressed.

On the first day of the eight-week group, twelve women sat in a circle in a large conference room with floor-to-ceiling glass walls. They introduced themselves and shared what had brought them to the group. It was an evening event, and the room buzzed with the residual energy of the day and the anticipation of what was to come.

Sheryl rushed in late from work. Her job was her main source of stress. She felt overworked and underappreciated and often fought with her boss. When she left work, she usually felt drained and irritable.

Delores, who rode the bus more than an hour to attend the group—there were no other mental health resources in her neighborhood—had spent the previous year as the primary caregiver for her ill mother, who had passed away a month earlier. During the time that her mother was sick, Delores gave all of her energy to caretaking. She stopped working, spending time with friends, and doing most all of the things that she enjoyed. In her words, she stopped living. She was consumed with her role as caregiver and gained more than fifty pounds in the process. Now she was coping with grief and loneliness and was struggling to find a new life's purpose.

Mary's twenty-seven-year-old son, her only child, had been murdered two years before in the neighborhood in which they lived. Every day that she walked outside her house was another reminder of her tragic and untimely loss.

For Gladys, the stress came from her husband. He was disabled, unemployed, angry, and drank heavily. She put all of her energy into him and complained that he didn't want to help himself.

The women who attended these mindfulness groups were of all different ages, backgrounds, and life experiences. The majority of them were single, heads of their households, and caring for multiple children or grandchildren. Just more than half had experienced a traumatic event, including witnessing the death of a loved one to gun violence, learning about the death of a child on the news, discovering a child who committed suicide by hanging, and physical and/or sexual assault. Almost a third of them suffered from PTSD.

The women came to the group feeling close to the edge and realized that they needed *something* to help them cope. Many of them felt helpless and like they had nowhere else to turn. Their families didn't listen to them or understand how they felt, and neither did doctors. Part of what made them feel safe coming to the group was seeing the face of a friendly Black woman (me) on the brochure. *Maybe she'll get it*, they thought.

The women needed practical skills to help them deal with their inner and outer worlds. One woman said, "During stressful periods of time, you kind of get the sky-is-falling type mentality, start running around, and I know that I need to stop feeling like that. It is just like the jack-in-the-box, na-na-na-na, and I feel like this bad thing is going to jump out of the box. I can't keep being scared all the time. I need something to help me get ready for whatever the next stressor may be in my life. I need something to gird me; it's the only way I'm gon' make it." The women needed to know that they weren't "crazy" and there was nothing "wrong" with them. Some came eagerly and others with hesitation and skepticism. Being in the group gave them a space where they could take off the mask of strength and be honest about what was really going on in their lives, without being judged or having the information used against them. Slowly, the load they were carrying by holding it all inside felt a little bit lighter. By seeking help, they felt more in control of themselves and their lives.

At the end of the group, Marjorie said: "We [Black women] are always superwomen and we have to be able to do everything and that brings out a lot of stress. This group helped me to reorganize and put things into the proper perspective and learn that I have an opportunity to learn how to calm myself down and recognize what is going on."

Marjorie had become more mindfully aware of her stressors and her automatic reactions to stress, and now she was able to use that awareness to choose a healthier behavioral response (versus automatic reaction) when stress confronted her. She developed the capacity to STOP—Stop, Take a Breath, Observe, and Proceed. Rather than panic or get angry when a stressor hit, now she could see the stressor coming, slow down, and respond with intention.

The women in the group learned not only how to deal with stress but also how to expand their view to notice the small moments of joy and pleasure that they were missing out on when they were singularly focused on stress. They learned to embrace these precious moments with gratitude. They became more aware of how thoughts of the past, worries for the future, and self-critical and guilt-ridden thoughts cause suffering. They learned how to be more compassionate, forgiving, and accepting of their true and full selves.

While they learned practical skills about mindfulness and stress management, they also were embedded in a safe space where they could be seen, heard, and understood. The other women in the group provided support and encouragement. Women who had been dealing with stress secretly and on their own no longer felt alone. Most of the women had never before participated in a stress-management group or had any mental health treatment. When the group was over, they left with a commitment to themselves to prioritize their mental and physical wellness.

FOURTEEN

Let Go and Let God

*B**ut by the grace of God I am what I am, and his grace toward me has not been in vain* (1 Cor 15:10, NRSV).

People who attend religious services more frequently are less likely to have a mental health condition (such as depression or anxiety) or substance abuse problem than those who attend less frequently.[1] Black women and men are more religious than Americans as a whole. According to the 2009 Pew Research Center *Religious Portrait of African-Americans*, 83 percent of Black adults (versus 61 percent of whites) say that they believe in God, 73 percent (versus 52 percent) say that they pray daily, and 47 percent (versus 34 percent) say that they attend religious services at least once a week.[2] The majority of Black adults (69 percent) report feeling a sense of spiritual peace and well-being. Although therapy has become more accessible and acceptable, religious practices and spiritual beliefs historically have been, and continue to be, an important part of emotional well-being for Black women.

African American religious culture was born of slavery.[3] The enslavement of diverse African people produced distinctive religious perspectives that helped individuals and communities to persevere under the dehumanization of slavery and gave them refuge from systematic oppression. The message of individual freedom and direct communication with God resonated deeply with enslaved people.

In the beginning of the eighteenth century, African Americans embraced Christianity and gathered in independent church communities. Churches provided places for spiritual support, educational opportunity, economic development, and political activism. African American religious institutions served as contexts in which African American people made meaning of the experience of enslavement. Religion and spirituality provided individual comfort, a means to endure the brutality of slavery, and a promise of salvation.

In their worship, the enslaved listened to Black preachers affirm their humanity. They could relate to the persecution of Jesus Christ and likened His crucifixion to the lynching of Black men. They found hope in the scriptural promises of a future without oppression. The biblical narrative of the exodus, when God delivered the Israelites out of slavery, offered African Americans the promise of God's deliverance of suffering people.

After the end of enslavement, African American Christians looked to the Bible for other sources of inspiration and knowledge about their future. Their religious practice expanded to encompass understanding other circumstances of suffering such as poverty, abuse, sickness, and loss. Attending worship service and Bible study gave Black people a way to conceptualize their struggles within the larger struggle between good and evil.[4]

We cling to the scripture that says, "We boast in our sufferings, knowing that suffering produces endurance, and endurance produces character, and character produces hope, and hope does not disappoint us, because God's love has been poured into our hearts through the Holy Spirit that has been given to us" (Rom 5:3–5, NRSV).

After the Civil War, the church focused on the spiritual, secular, and political concerns of the Black community. It was at the center of the civil rights movement. The Black church was one of the few places where Black people could experience power and prestige and the respect otherwise denied them by predominantly white institutions.

Although men still hold most of the traditional leadership roles within the church, such as pastor, the church has been a place for Black women to be lifted up and affirmed in their leadership positions. Furthermore, Black women within independent Black church denominations have always constituted the majority of members and have been active contributors to the church, serving as fundraisers, evangelists, missionaries, and mothers of the church.

This tradition among Black women of using faith in God to gather their strength to get through difficult times is a core part of being a strong Black woman. The belief in an all-knowing, all-powerful God was passed down to me from my grandmother and my mother, just as it has been passed down among generations of Black women.

When I was a little girl, Grandma would get into her big blue Cadillac on Sunday mornings, slowly back it out of the garage, and glide up the hill to Lilydale Progressive Church to thank Jesus for all that he had done for her.

On the car radio, Rev. Paul Jones crooned:

I've had some good days
I've had some hills to climb

I've had some weary days
And some sleepless nights
But when I look around
And I think things over
All of my good days
Outweigh my bad days
I won't complain

When Grandma walked through the church doors, her aura
preceded her. In this sacred space, she received the respect that she
knew she was inherently entitled to receive. The familiar congregants quieted and sat up a little straighter. She greeted sisters so-
and-so from a distance with pursed lips, slight nods, and modest
waves. Left of center, fourth row on the aisle, she sat upright and
dignified, in direct sight of the pastor.

Being at church, in God's presence, must have given her a
slight reprieve from her trials and tribulations. The safety people
rest in when they have faith that they are guarded and protected.
The comfort they feel when they are nakedly seen and known. The
freedom they capture when they lay their burdens down. Grandma
carried the Word with her wherever she went, as her armor, ready
to use as needed.

Grandma was a good and faithful Christian servant, someone whom the pastor could hold up as an example. On Saturday
nights, she sat at the kitchen table in the basement in her housecoat
with her Bible and Sunday School teacher's guide in front of her,
underlining scripture and making notes as she diligently prepared
the lesson for the next day. After Sunday School, she asserted her
position in the center aisle as head of the usher board and made
sure that proceedings ran with order. As chair of the women's day

committee, she put together a program designed to inspire souls to the highest standards.

For Easter, she dressed me in delicate and sophisticated ensembles, complete with hat, lace gloves, and shiny white patent leather shoes, that conveyed with certainty my virtue and, by default, hers. She reveled in pride on the Sundays that I accompanied her to church, one of the few occasions you could truly see her exhale joy. I was the embodiment of her dreams.

When I was seven years old, I was baptized at the Mount Moriah Missionary Baptist Church by the Reverend O. C. Nicks. Rev. Nicks was like a Black Santa Claus—tall and heavyset, with a big, round, protruding belly that held up the gold chains he wore on top of his pitch-black church suits. His few remaining strands of thin, greasy, wavy hair were combed over the wide bald spot in the middle of his head.

When my Sunday School teacher told him that I had professed to my Sunday School class that I believed in my heart that Jesus died for my sins, was buried, and on the third day rose from the dead so that I would be saved, his twinkling eyes looked down on me and he smiled. He placed his thick, jewel-adorned fingers on top of my head and prayed. Something about his soft, warm hand on my head settled my spirit.

"Bless this child, oh Lord!" he prayed. "Watch over her and keep her safe. Bless her mother, oh Lord, so that she may guide her baby girl in your Word. These prayers we ask in the name of the Father, the Son, and the Holy Spirit. Let the church say amen. Amen. Amen. Amen, again!"

Three weeks later, my mom and dad, grandmother, godmother, and a few close family friends came to the church in the evening to hear me again confess my belief and see Rev. Nicks baptize me. The mothers of the church fussed over me, dressing me in a white robe and head wrap. The event was ceremonial, and although I didn't fully understand its significance at the time, I knew it was to be taken seriously.

After I had been prepared, I walked up the hideaway stairs behind the choir stand to the wading pool that had been filled with cool water. Rev. Nicks was already standing in the pool, and he took my hand to guide me down the stairs. Then he placed his hands firmly on my shoulders and asked, "Do you believe that Jesus is the son of God?"

"Yes," I replied.

"Do you believe that he died for your sins, was buried, and on the third day rose from the grave?"

"Yes."

"Do you accept him as your Lord and savior?"

"Yes."

"Inger, my child, I now baptize you in the name of the Father, the Son, and the Holy Ghost!"

I pinched my nose, and he dunked me back for a full submersion into the water. I came up trembling and gasping for air. My sins had been washed away, and I was saved.

"Hallelujah!" Grandma shouted. My mom's eyes teared up. My dad nodded in slight approval. There was a felt sense of both joy and relief in knowing that now, when I went out into the world, I would be protected by the blood of Jesus and saved from eternal damnation. After the ceremony was complete, we went to the dining hall in the basement and had fried chicken and pound cake to celebrate.

My spirituality has given me direction in times of uncertainty, strength in moments of fear and hopefulness when the future looked bleak. It surrounds me in a community of steadfast believers and prayer warriors who collectively guarantee that God's mighty plans to bless me will be revealed and that suffering today will not compare to the glory that is to come.

My mother texts me devotionals every day that remind me to stay centered on my faith in God rather than worldly distractions that can produce angst and despair. When she sent scripture that read, "Trust in the Lord with all your heart, do not lean on your own insight" (Prov 3:5), I was reminded to "let go and let God" and not get caught up in the anxiety-producing dysfunction of my worry-thoughts. When I am restless that things aren't going my way, on my time, I remind myself to have faith that God ultimately will give me the desires of my heart.

Given historical context and the generational importance of the Black church, it is deeply engrained in Black culture that any problems we face are to be handled by God. Many Black people believe that spiritual beliefs and practices, particularly prayer, are an important part of coping with illness, that they promote healing, and that God is ultimately responsible for mental, physical, and spiritual health.[5]

The types of issues people go to clergy for help with include grief, family conflict, marital problems, and parenting challenges. Clergy provide help in the form of prayer, reading the Bible, listening, advice, comfort/sympathy, and advocating on their behalf.[6] Counsel is usually sought only if the problems are so severe that people feel like they are going to have a "nervous breakdown." People who first seek help from clergy are less likely to later seek other types of professional mental health treatment.[7]

Black people tend to consider aspects related to their spirituality, such as having faith in God, being able to ask God for forgiveness, and prayer, the most important part of their depression treatment.[8] Among those Black people with a diagnosed mental health condition, 63 percent use prayer or spiritual practices to cope with their condition. In a study of more than a thousand Black women, depression was the condition most commonly treated with religion/spirituality.[9]

My client Gloria was able to integrate her spiritual beliefs with therapy as a part of her healing. God has always been at the center of Gloria's life. God is evident in every word that she speaks and every step that she takes. Sundays are sacred, and she never allows anything to interfere with this time to praise and worship God. Gloria has been an active member of her church for the past thirty years, serving in various church roles, attending Sunday school, multiple services, Bible class, and volunteering regularly.

Her designation as deaconess reminds her that she is somebody of worth, dignity, and respect. She sits in the front row in her white suit with pride. No matter what has happened during the week, when she leaves church on Sunday, she feels restored and renewed. Instead of her children, with whom she has had strained relationships, her church family is her family, her core group of friends, her prayer warriors, and her primary support system.

When Gloria felt down, she would reach out to her prayer group and simply tell them she was "going through," and they prayed for her. Despite not outwardly expressing her challenges, she internalized the word of God. "God never said that we weren't going to go through anything," she maintains. "But his strength is made perfect in my weakness."

Although Gloria feels deeply embedded in her church community, they know only one side of her—the strong side that always shows up with a smile on her face. They know nothing of her experiences with childhood sexual abuse, domestic violence, fractured relationships with her children, financial worries, depression, anxiety, and traumatic stress—all of which she battles regularly.

Gloria was ashamed to tell her church friends that she was in therapy. She believed that they would judge her and think that she had lost her faith in God. Older Black adults are more likely to believe that depression occurs because of a loss of faith; therefore, regaining faith through prayer, talking to a pastor, and going to church is the only way to heal, making them less likely to pursue traditional mental health care.[10] Gloria quietly resists that notion and says to me, "I know that God sent you here to help me. I know you can't say it, but I know that you love me too."

Gloria integrates the strategies that she has learned in therapy with her spiritual beliefs. She uses scripture for *cognitive restructuring*—a process whereby together we identify and dispute irrational negative thoughts. For instance, when she has the thought *Nobody loves me*, she reminds herself, *God loves me, and he said I'm never alone*. She has become aware of her "stinking thinking" and rejects it when it shows up.

Every morning she reads her Bible and listens to her gospels to keep herself immersed in the Word. The Word of God gives her guidance, comfort, and encouragement and shifts the focus from thoughts of herself to the Holy Spirit. This daily practice gets each day started on the right foot.

In the past when Gloria became anxious, she would start shaking, pacing, and frantically calling friends until someone picked up or she burst out into a crying spell. Now she pulls to mind a verse from scripture such as, *Be still and know that I am God*. She pauses and prays that the Lord bring her peace. Her worry subsides because she believes wholeheartedly that God will provide for and take care of her. "You can worry, or you can pray, but you can't do both," she tells me.

When she doesn't have enough money to get by, she prays that God will make a way, and God always does. When she didn't know how she was going to get back and forth to work, she received a call that she had been approved for a reduced-fare bus card. When she didn't know how she was going to pay her electricity bill, the sisters at the church ordered three dozen of her homemade butter cookies and gave her a $20 tip. When she thought that her social security disability might get taken away because she worked over the allowable number of hours, she said, "God, if this is what you have for me, I know you'll make a way."

God showed up, not only for Gloria's finances, but also in her personal life. After years of praying that God heal the hearts of her estranged children and bring the family together again, they gradually started reaching out and calling her more. They attended her birthday party and invited her to Thanksgiving and Christmas dinner. When she showed me the pictures of them all together, she could barely contain her excitement.

Research has found that prayer is psychologically beneficial for people who see God as loving, as Gloria does. People who focus their prayers on being thankful for what they have and expressing concern for others tend to be less depressed. Studies have shown that the negative health effects of financial problems, which Black people are susceptible to, are reduced among people who pray regularly for others. The more that people pray, the less likely they are to engage in unhealthy behaviors such as drug and alcohol use. Additionally, prayer helps people to focus their attention and reduces the extent to which they are distracted by negative emotions. Finally, prayer has been found to be strongly connected to the value of sacrifice, which is a core aspect of being a strong Black woman.[11]

Although Black women lean on their religious practices and spiritual beliefs for guidance and comfort during difficult times, they are unlikely to seek direct counsel from their pastors for extremely personal issues. Problems such as child abuse, domestic violence, infidelity, sexuality, depression, suicidal thoughts, and drug addiction are often not openly discussed within the Black church. While these issues may be prevalent among churchgoers, and there is an unspoken recognition that they exist, few are willing to discuss them in a church environment.

Pastors who have close relationships with their members are uniquely positioned to notice emotional and behavioral changes in their congregants. They may observe that a member hasn't been attending service as much, isn't as involved on committees as she used to be, or doesn't have the sense of joy that she used to have. This trusted relationship can provide a critical gateway for faith leaders to refer their members to specialized mental health, domestic violence, or substance abuse treatment.

Undoubtedly, church has many benefits for spiritual and emotional health. The church is a free space for people who are suffering to come as they are and be received with open arms. It is a place where they can sit in the back and receive the word of God without being put on the spot. At the same time, individual support and counsel are also available, if desired.

The lessons given in church instruct us how to live a meaningful life, make it through the difficult times, and find meaning in trials and tribulations. The Word of God gives specific instructions on how to cope with difficult emotions and find peace. Church is a place where we can go and be lifted up and redeemed from life's mistakes, knowing that we are unconditionally loved by God and are never alone.

FIFTEEN

Self-Care Is Not Selfish

My grandmother's model as a strong Black woman has had tremendous influence over my life. She passed down to me her ambition, perseverance, faith in God, and pure hustle. From her I learned well how to take care of myself and not *need* anyone for anything. Her legacy has given me a sense of pride, purpose, and responsibility. When I am out in the world, I hold my head up high in the dignified, self-assured way that she taught me.

However, I also understand how the strength that was ingrained in me early on can get in the way of my showing up and living fully. In the past, my strength has been a cover for my insecurities. It has protected me from the negative judgments I feared from other people if they knew the truth about my family, my relationships, and the intense emotions that I felt. The suspicious and distrusting eye of my strength has held me back in conversations. It's kept me from sharing my ideas, boldly speaking my truth, and taking action. My strength has lied to me and told me that I had to put up with situations that didn't serve me because *I'm not a quitter* and *It's fine.* My strength has exhausted me and burned me out by convincing me that I had to do everything on my own. It made me believe that I don't need other people, when really I do. But, no more. Not today. Now I know that my strength is in my vulnerability.

In order to move away from being the kind of strong Black women who are merely surviving rather than thriving, we must embrace both our strengths and vulnerabilities and give ourselves permission to be human rather than expect to be superhuman. That means pulling back the mask of strength and showing the world the beauty in the core essence of our being.

What would it be like to rip the Band-Aid off and breathe air into your wounds? What parts of yourself have you been denying or holding back? When you are all alone, in stillness, not executing your role of partner, mother, or employee, without the things that you may use to cover yourself—house, car, clothes—who are you *really*? Imagine how it would feel to receive a hand of love and understanding and feel the warmth of that hand's support.

Starting today, let's give ourselves permission to be free to exist in a way that is not defined by the expectations of others. I invite you to stop trying to force yourself into being something that doesn't fit and allow yourself to just *be*. When we pretend to be someone other than who we really are, by denying or avoiding the impact that our experiences have had on us, we not only discount our individual humanity, but we disconnect ourselves from others.

The first step in the journey from suffering toward healing is to identify the sources of your suffering and how that pain shows up in your life. Then you must accept (rather than deny) your complex experiences *as they are*, without shame or judgment, but with compassion. Let go of the self-deprecating stories that you have told yourself about who you are and why your life *is what it is*. Free yourself of the agony rooted in the past that you have been hold-ing on to and know that it does not serve you. Bring awareness to your triggers in the moment, name the trigger and the feeling, and respond mindfully rather than react impulsively. This is how we honor the full range of our feelings and also manage our emotions in a healthy way.

For example, you can bring awareness to the fact that when you feel down, you start to think about all of the things that aren't going right in life, and you stop answering the phone and instead snug-gle down on the couch with Netflix and ice cream, which makes you feel worse. But instead, when you're headed down that familiar dark road, you can embody a sense of gratitude for the goodness that is present in your life and do something that might bring you joy—like call a friend, color in a mindfulness coloring book, or step outside for some air. If you take the steps to change the behavior, the feelings will follow.

Although there may be aspects of your circumstances that you aren't able to change right away, you can take steps to change how you think, feel, and behave. Even as the chaos of the world con-tinues to cyclone around you, you alone are responsible for your own emotions. Take a moment to identify what is in your control, and what isn't, and work with that which is within your control to create incremental positive behavioral changes. This kind of inten-tional caring for ourselves can feel like a luxury, even exorbitant. But in the words of author Audre Lorde, "Caring for myself is not self-indulgence. It is self-preservation, and that is an act of political warfare."

Ladies, it's time for us to armor up so we can be our best selves. We as Black women generally have not given ourselves permis-sion to focus on our own healing. But it's time for us to resist the conditioned urge to constantly sacrifice our wellness and unabashedly prioritize taking care of ourselves. In addition to seeking the help of a mental health provider, here are a few behavioral strategies that you can use every day on your own to improve your mood, well-being, and daily life functioning.

Get dressed. When you are depressed, sometimes it can be difficult to function normally. You may feel the urge to withdraw, spend more time in bed, and escape from the world. When you stay in bed all day without getting dressed, you can end up feeling more sluggish, and in turn, more down. In these moments, maintain the basic daily self-care practices of getting out of bed, showering, and getting dressed each day, even when you don't feel like it. The mere act of letting warm water touch your body and inhaling the scent of soap can help you feel more awake and alive.

Maintain a routine. When you are feeling stressed, you may notice that your daily schedule falls by the wayside. Suddenly you're staying up late at night, sleeping in later in the morning, and maybe even taking multiple naps throughout the day. Go to bed and wake up at the same time every day. Establishing a regular sleep/wake routine can help to stabilize your mood. Create a calendar of activities that includes obligations such as work, errands, social activities, or just quiet time to yourself. Shut off electronic devices at least an hour before bed to help slow the mind down and prepare for rest. Make sure the routine that you set is realistic and manageable enough so that you can maintain it.

Do the things that bring you joy. When people are down or depressed, they deny themselves even the opportunity for pleasure by saying to themselves, "I'll do it when I feel better." But it is the *doing* that will make you feel better! Try to do something that brings you joy, no matter how small, each day. It might be having a good cup of coffee in the morning, going for a short walk at lunch, watching your favorite TV show in the evening, listening to music, getting lost in a book, calling a friend on the phone, snuggling with your partner, watching your child play, journaling, coloring, cooking, gardening. Whatever it is, do something for *you*.

Create space. When you lead a busy life, you can get caught in the cycle of doing all the time. Your schedule can easily become packed with a long to-do list, and you're constantly running from one thing to the next. This busyness can trick you into thinking that you're being productive, when actually it may just be serving as a distraction from the unrest within.

Take time to create space in your day. Allow yourself a few minutes, five, ten, or fifteen, to just *be*. You may take ten minutes to lie mindfully in bed in the morning before getting up, noticing your breath, the sensations of your body, the contents of your mind. Or you might take ten minutes in stillness at the end of the day to just be quiet and breathe. This space allows you the opportunity to notice the thoughts and feelings that are showing up—even those that might be uncomfortable. This could also be a time that you use for prayer or meditation. Take advantage of this opportunity to connect with your innermost self. By creating space to just be, you can free yourself from the things that are weighing you down and actually be more present and productive.

Eat mindfully. If you aren't keeping a schedule, your eating habits can become chaotic too. Pay attention to your internal cues for hunger. Plan your meals and snacks in advance. Try to take time to savor and enjoy your meals, rather than rushing through them while multitasking. If you're going to have a steak, or a good burger, slow down long enough to really enjoy it. Rather than eating your lunch at your desk as you work, or skipping it entirely, perhaps find a space to eat outside. Eat foods that give you sustainable energy, such as fruits, vegetables, legumes, and whole grains rather than high-fat and carbohydrate-laden fast foods, which can contribute to fatigue, sluggishness, and ill health.

With food often comes alcohol. Pay attention to increases in your alcohol intake during times of stress. Limit how much alcohol you drink, and find other ways to self-soothe, such as drinking de-caffeinated tea, taking a warm bath, listening to music, doing gentle yoga, or meditating.

Set manageable goals and expectations. Sometimes stress is driven by the unrealistic expectations that we put on ourselves. You may convince yourself that, after completing a demanding day at work and then going home and cooking and caring for your children, it is also necessary to make sure the house is perfectly clean. You might take on another volunteer project or start planning an elaborate birthday party. What's worse, you persuade yourself that all of these things *must* be done right now. Take it easy on yourself. Give yourself some grace. Identify what is a necessity, what would be nice, and what is entirely unnecessary.

Pay attention to your thoughts. Our feelings are closely connected to our thoughts, which ultimately shape our behavior. Notice when you are getting stuck in patterns of unhealthy, dysfunctional thinking. People who are depressed often have an automatic negative tape of self-blame, guilt, shame, and regret that plays in their minds. The tape may say things like *I should have told someone sooner that I was being molested*; *I don't deserve this job because I'm not as smart as the people around me*; *I'm a failure*; *I'm pathetic*; and *Nobody loves me*. Notice when you are putting yourself down and being overly critical of yourself. Reframe these negative thoughts and develop a new, judgment-free internal dialogue.

Instead, you might say to yourself, *I'm taking the necessary steps to confront my trauma now*; *If I weren't qualified for this job, I wouldn't be here*; *I'm doing the best that I can*; *I don't have to be perfect*; and *I'm loved.*

Practice self-compassion. Often, we are our own worst critics. When we are going through a difficult time, we can beat ourselves up with shoulda, woulda, couldas. Practice talking to yourself with the same kindness, warmth, and understanding that you would offer to a friend. Although you may feel all alone, know that moments of suffering are a natural part of the human experience. No one is perfect, everyone makes mistakes. That's what makes us human. Take a step back so that you can observe your emotions clearly rather than getting lost in them, and keep them in perspective given everything else that is happening in your life.

Look through the wide lens. When people are depressed, they tend to have tunnel vision—they see only the things that aren't going right in life. Depressed people tend to minimize the positive and exaggerate the negative. They see only the father who abandoned them, the relationship that they lost, the promotion that they didn't get, the money they don't have, the kid who keeps getting into trouble. Take the blinders off. Expand your vision to notice and hold space for everything in the picture. In doing so, you may also see things for which you can be grateful, such as the friends who stepped up to comfort you after the breakup, the other recognitions that you received at work, or the sweet snuggles that your baby girl gives at the end of the day.

Have clear and measurable goals. When people set goals for self-improvement, they are often big and lofty, such as "be more happy" or "make more money" or "lose more weight" or "spend more time with family." These big goals ultimately lead them to feel more overwhelmed and defeated when they aren't met. It's important that the goals you set are SMART—that is, Specific, Manageable, Attainable, Relevant, and Time-bound.

When Gloria noticed that she had been gaining some of the weight back that she lost after surgery, she set a goal to exercise more and eat fewer sweets. In therapy, we refined her goal to make it more specific: she planned to go to the gym in her apartment building and walk on the treadmill for twenty minutes once a week, work out in her apartment using a video for twenty minutes once a week, and stop buying pastries on her way to work in the morning. Break down larger goals into smaller, time-specific fragments. Congratulate yourself for each small success.

Set an intention. While goals are focused on the future and have a specific result in mind, intentions are lived each day, independent of any particular outcome. Set an intention for how you want to show up each day. Here are some examples:

> *I invite myself to experience more ease.*
> *I will allow myself to experience joy and pleasure.*
> *I will give myself the space to slow down and rest.*
> *I will show up as my full self.*
> *Every day I will treat myself and others with kindness.*

Write the intention down, then let it go. Release yourself from any attachment to a specific outcome. Know that intentions are lived moment by moment.

Reach out to your support system. When things aren't going right, you might feel the urge to withdraw from friends and family. You stop answering the phone, you stop going to church, or you start skipping your exercise class. Maybe you don't want anyone to know what's going on with you. The thought of having to answer questions feels like torture. Perhaps your relationship is on the rocks, you're having financial troubles, or you simply feel depleted by all that you have to do. A wise person on Instagram once said, "Behind every successful woman there's a group text hypin' her up." This is the village of women that we rely on for support, prayer, and advice. They share information and resources. They provide help shuttling kids around and babysitting when needed. They drive each other to doctors' appointments. They go to movies, dinner, and church together. Research has shown that people with strong social support networks are happier, healthier, and live longer. Identify the positive people in your life, and nurture these relationships. Allow yourself to be vulnerable with those whom you trust, and ask for help when you need it.

Exercise. The mind and body are intricately connected. Suffering of the mind shows up in the body, and taking good care of the body benefits the mind. Aerobic exercise, such as jogging, swimming, cycling, walking, gardening, and dancing, have been shown to reduce mild to moderate anxiety and depression. These improvements in mood are due to reducing physiological reactivity to stress. Physical activity can center the mind, improve self-efficacy and self-esteem, and promote social interaction, all of which contribute to better mental health.

Exercise protects against a number of chronic health conditions, such as obesity, diabetes, and cardiovascular disease. Exercise can also increase energy and stamina and improve sleep quality. The Centers for Disease Control and Prevention recommends that each week adults do at least 150 minutes of moderate-intensity aerobic activity (such as brisk walking) or 75 minutes of vigorous activity (such as running or swimming laps).[1] You may start by building ten to fifteen minutes of exercise into your day. Take the stairs at work rather than the elevator, or take a walk during your lunch hour. You may also find an exercise buddy to keep you accountable to your workout goals.

Don't forget to breathe. Stress, anxiety, and trauma can literally come for your breath. When you are under stress, it can feel like your heart is thumping out of your chest, your throat is closing in, and you are gasping for air. In these moments of acute stress, stop what you're doing and be still. Notice the sensations in your body. Bring your awareness to your breath. To start, don't try to change it in any way; just allow it to be as it is. Notice the air coming in through your nose, moving down to your lungs, and filling your abdomen. Feel your belly expand out with every inhale and drop down with every exhale. If you notice your breath getting stuck in your chest, draw the air in and down to your belly. Ride the wave of each and every breath. Inhale, exhale. Inhale, exhale. Feel the breath expand throughout your body to your limbs, reminding you that you are present and alive. Your breath is your anchor, a place that you can always come back to.

Although trauma has been pervasive among Black women for generations, it does not represent the entirety of our human experience. Even within the trauma, we have a remarkable capacity for healing and joy. Healing is passed down in the wisdom of our ancestors. It is the abundant and overbearing love that we find in community with our grandmothers, mothers, aunties, and friends. It wraps around us, holds us tight, and comforts us. Healing comes in speaking our truth and allowing our stories to be told. It is standing firmly in our authentic selves. It is allowing ourselves to be in community with each other and receive support. It is the wild and brilliant flame of strength that eternally endures inside of us.

Joy does not deny or minimize the reality of the painful experiences that we may have endured or require that we silence our pain. Joyful moments are hiding in the crevices of our lives, waiting to be seen and held tenderly.

SIXTEEN

Joy Comes in the Morning

After I ended the relationship with Nathan, I poured all of the time and energy that I had been giving to him into my own emotional wellness. It seemed like a good time to start using on myself the behavioral activation strategies that I'd learned in graduate school and was teaching to others. *Behavioral activation* is a type of therapy in which you intentionally schedule enjoyable activities and opportunities to connect with other people, since when you're depressed or anxious, you're more likely to withdraw and less likely to do the things that you enjoy.

I set a goal to run on a treadmill five days a week for one hour. I was not a runner, but I wanted to be, and I needed something positive to focus my mind on. I couldn't afford to join a health club, so I went to the small, dingy, but free gym in my apartment complex.

The first few weeks I could barely run five minutes before something rose up in my body, punched me in the chest, and left me heaving for air. My tingling, itching, and wobbly legs stood in stark contrast with the fresh workout gear that I'd purchased for the challenge. I thought I was *strong* and in shape—well, at least strong enough to run longer than five minutes. Despite failing to meet my own expectations, my mind and body felt good, so I kept going. I walked for a few minutes, caught my breath, and then built up the courage to run again. *Run, walk. Walk, run.*

On Sundays, the gospel show *Joyful Noise* played on the old fuzzy television in the corner and gave me an extra boost. I could feel my spirit lifting. *Run, walk. Walk, run.* Eventually, the running segments became longer than the walking segments. One evening three months later, I snatched off the towel covering the time on the treadmill after two thirty-minute TV shows had passed, and it read 1:04. I had done it!

Around the same time, I reconnected with yoga. I had practiced it off and on since college, but it had been years since I had attended a class. Now that the relationship with Nathan was over, I had a lot of free time on my hands. Rather than sulk, I ran during the week and went to yoga on the weekends.

Initially, I saw my yoga practice as another physical workout. When I nailed difficult poses, I felt like I was on top of the world. I was *doing*. Doing something for myself made me feel good. Therapy, running, and yoga (and a break from men) were my first steps toward healing.

Years after I ended my relationship with Nathan, I am still deeply engaged in my yoga practice. It is a key part of my emotional and physical wellness. As I practiced with teachers who taught yoga sutras—teachings on the theory and practice of yoga—and incorporated mindfulness into the practice, I noticed my mind become more at ease.

Yoga gave me a time and space at least twice a week to embrace stillness and check in with the contents of my mind and the sensations of my body. I learned to be *in the present moment* rather than focusing on the guilt and regret of the past, which was gone, or worry about the future, which was yet to come. Every beat of my heart, every inhale and exhale, marks where I am, right now.

Yoga taught me to accept things as they are in the present, not where they were in the past or as I might wish them to be in the future. Despite how much I may want to do that inversion or balancing pose and believe that I "should" be able to do it by now since I have been practicing for so long, I must accept that it is not where I am right now. Where I am is standing in this room, with two feet planted firmly on the ground, alive and breathing. And that is enough.

This way of being present relieves us of the burden of our past and allows our world to open up to take in the goodness that is available right now. It gives us the power to see more fully and clearly without focusing on only the suffering. With each moment that we live in the past, we lose the opportunity to enjoy the present or create a new future. The present moment is the only moment that is truly available to us and the only moment over which we have some control.

Through yoga I noticed how my breath became shallow and rapid when I felt anxious. I learned how to slow my breath down and breathe into the spaces of discomfort. I became more kind and patient and learned to let go of rigid expectations for myself and others or situations that don't serve me. As I became more physically flexible in my yoga practice, I became more emotionally flexible in life and able to adjust to the unexpected life challenges that inevitably come. When things didn't go my way, I didn't get as upset as I used to. Most important, yoga taught me to trust my intuition. I became more confident in listening to that inner voice rather than the distracting chatter of the world around me.

Yoga has been vitally important in helping me to cope with daily stress and anxiety and also is an integral part of my therapy practice. I'm one of those people who schedules plans around my yoga class, and I can feel the difference in my mood and body if I miss a class. Several research studies have shown that practicing yoga has a wide range of physical and mental health benefits, including reducing stress, depression, anxiety, blood pressure, heart rate, muscle pain, and headaches.[1] Yoga also improves sleep, attention, concentration, and overall well-being. Although not commonly known, Black women activists like Rosa Parks and Angela Davis used yoga as a part of their wellness practice. They realized that it was necessary to be mentally and physically well in order to effectively carry out their work. Since the seventies, healers like Krishna Kaur, master meditation and yoga teacher; and Queen Afua, holistic health expert, have been teaching on the benefits of meditation and yoga for healing from trauma. While the majority of yoga practitioners are white, more and more Black women are walking intentionally toward, or stumbling upon, yoga for their healing. Chelsea Jackson Roberts, Jessamyn Stanley, Crystal McCreary, and Sara Clark have redefined the face of yoga, and in doing so they have inspired thousands of Black women to step onto the mat.

A few years ago I decided that I wanted to deepen my foundational knowledge and practice of yoga so I did a 250-hour yoga teacher training program. The summer after I completed the training, I traveled to the Kripalu Center for Yoga and Health in Stockbridge, Massachusetts, for a Black yoga teacher's retreat. As soon as I arrived at the retreat space, which sits on a hilltop in the Berkshires surrounded by more than a hundred acres of woodlands, hills, valleys, and Lake Mahkeenac, I felt the textured presence of dozens of Black women of all ages from across the country who abundantly occupied a place known for its whiteness.

On the second day of the retreat, I sat in a dignified cross-legged position in a circle with more than sixty other women waiting for a session on yoga and sound healing to begin as the midafternoon sun beamed its light on all of us. The instructor, Chante, from Washington, DC, sat in the middle dressed all in white, adorned in colorful jewelry, surrounded by seven white singing bowls of various sizes. She started the session by sharing that she was introduced to yoga at a time in her life when she was suffering. After her father's death, she had a hard time shaking her deep grief, and a friend invited her to a yoga class. She acknowledged that yoga was just the first step in her journey toward healing from the grief of losing her father, other relationships, and expectations of what should have or could have been.

Then she asked that each one of us name one thing that we wanted to let go of in order to make room for something else. One by one women gave voice to their afflictions, naming all the issues we face in addition to being burdened by other people's expectations, putting other people's needs first, long to-do lists, and holding on to people or things that don't serve us. Each burden that was offered was held with seeing eyes, nods of the head, and validating shouts of *Ase!*

We all claimed our healing in harmony. We wanted to be free of everything that troubled us and wore us down to make room for joy, forgiveness, kindness, compassion, acceptance, stillness, connection, love, truth, creativity, lightness, confidence, and our voice saying *Yes* to alignment with purpose and the voice of God.

After the last woman spoke, Chante asked us to stand up in the circle, shoulder to shoulder. "If you have a hurt that you've been carrying for at least a year, take a deep inhale, exhale, and scream to let it go," she said. The room roared.

"If you have a hurt that you've been carrying for at least five years, take a deep inhale, exhale, and scream to let it go." The room roared even louder, and I felt the energetic vibration run through my body.

"If you have a hurt that you've been carrying for at least ten years, take an inhale, exhale, and then release it all." The room collectively expelled decades of generational suffering. Tears rolled down my face and my body trembled. We stood together in silence, seeing and being seen. Understanding and being understood. Feeling the exuberant liberation of letting go. The pervasiveness of the burdens that Black women carry, interlaced within their resilient joy, was sobering.

Strong and . . .

I am a strong Black woman
My past struggles do not define me
The future is mine to take hold of
I release myself of guilt, regret, shame, fear, and worry
I have known suffering, but I have the capacity to heal
I surrender to my innermost divine power
And affirmatively claim my truth
Holding all parts of myself in loving-
kindness, compassion, and peace
Always knowing
I am enough
Just as I am

Acknowledgments

I am thankful to God for making the dream of this book come true. Thank you to my mother and grandmother, my first examples of strong Black women. You are my role models and inspiration. Thank you for every prayer that you prayed and the sacrifices that you made for me. Mother, I am propelled by your unconditional love and support. Thank you for courageously sharing our family story with me and allowing me to tell it. Grandma, I carry your legacy with great pride.

Thank you to my dad, who taught me so much about being strong in a challenging world, not caring what other people think, and always encouraged me to write. Thank you to my brother, Mat, for supporting this effort from the very beginning.

To my agent, Andrew, I am so grateful that you found me. Because of you, the loose idea of a book became a reality. Your guidance and wisdom have been invaluable throughout this process. To my editor, Tracy, thank you for helping to grow my vision and shape the story. I have cherished our many conversations and being able to exchange thoughts and real experiences with you. Thank you for holding and molding these words with such great care. To the entire Amistad and HarperCollins team, thank you for your help in making this book the best that it could be.

To my writing community, Natalie Moore, Sara Connell, Michele Weldon, and Marla Paul, thank you for helping me to believe that I could be a writer and for giving me tricks of the trade along the way.

To my clients, thank you for trusting me with your innermost thoughts. Though I am here for you to offer support and skills, you teach me so much. I hope always to be able to create a safe space for you to show up as your true selves and heal. I care for you deeply.

To the beloved friends whose stories are represented in this book, thank you for your courage and vulnerability in sharing your stories with me. You have given me, and the world, an amazing gift so that we might all see the beautifully complex women who walk among us each day. I pray that I have done you justice. I am forever indebted to you.

To the many other beautiful Black women whom I turn to for advice, mentorship, and encouragement, thank you. My village of sister-friends—Erin, Jackie, Melissa, Steffani, Auyana, Aminah, Kai, Kenyetta, Faith, Eni, Ny, Fanta, Rachel Y., Keisha, Michelle, TaShawna, Merci, Kim Foxx, Kennise, Auntie, Camille, The Ladies of Impact, my LGC Sistas, and so many others—thank you for lifting me up and holding me down. I love you forever.

And, to my beloved partner Ammon Ra, thank you for your unwavering support and encouragement.

Notes

ONE. I Am a Strong Black Woman

1 N. N. Watson and C. D. Hunter, "'I Had to Be Strong': Tensions in the Strong Black Woman Schema." *Journal of Black Psychology*, 2016. 42(5): 424–452.

2 "Black Americans: A Profile." Statistical Brief, US Department of Commerce Economics and Statistics Administration, Bureau of the Census, March 1993. https://www.census.gov/prod/1/statbrief/sb93_2.pdf.

3 Table 322.20, "Bachelor's degrees conferred by postsecondary institutions by race/ethnicity and sex of student," in *120 Years of American Education: A Statistical Portrait*. National Center for Education Statistics, US Department of Education, Office of Educational Research and Improvement, January 1993. https://nces.ed.gov/programs/digest/d16/tables/dt16_322.20.asp?current=yes.

TWO. On My Last Nerve

1 *Stress in America Report.* American Psychological Association, November 9, 2010. https://www.apa.org/news/press/releases/stress/2010/national-report.pdf.

2 Nina Banks, "Black Women's Labor Market History Reveals Deep-Seated Race and Gender Discrimination." Economic Policy Institute, Working Economics Blog, February 19, 2019. https://www.epi.org/blog/black-womens-labor-market -history-reveals-deep-seated-race-and-gender-discrimination/.

3 Ariane Hegewisch and Heidi Hartmann, "The Gender Wage Gap: 2018 Earnings Differences by Race and Ethnicity." Institute for Women's Policy Research, March 7, 2019. https:// iwpr.org/iwpr-general/the-gender-wage-gap-2018-earnings -differences-by-race-and-ethnicity/.

4 Ariane Hegewisch and Valerie Lacarte, "Breadwinner Mothers by Race/Ethnicity." Institute for Women's Policy Research, May 8, 2020. https://iwpr.org/iwpr-issues/race-ethnicity-gender -and-economy/breadwinner-mothers-by-race-ethnicity/.

5 "Degrees Conferred by Race and Sex." National Center for Education Statistics, Fast Facts, 2017. https://nces.ed.gov /fastfacts/display.asp?id=72.

6 "Barriers and Bias: The Status of Women in Leadership." American Association of University Women, 2017. https:// www.aauw.org/resources/research/barrier-bias/.

7 Asha DuMonthier, Chandra Childers, and Jessica Milli, "The Status of Black Women in the United States." Institute for Women's Policy Research, June 7, 2017. https://iwpr.org /iwpr-issues/race-ethnicity-gender-and-economy/the-status -of-black-women-in-the-united-states/.

8 American Psychological Association, *Stress in America: The Impact of Discrimination*. Stress in America Survey, March 10, 2016. https://www.apa.org/news/press/releases/stress/2015 /impact-of-discrimination.pdf.

9 R. A. Donovan et al., "Impact of Racial Macro- and Micro-

aggressions in Black Women's Lives: A Preliminary Analysis." *Journal of Black Psychology*, 2013. 39(2): 185–196.

10 I. Burnett-Zeigler, K. M. Bohnert, and M. Ilgen, "Ethnic Identity, Acculturation and the Prevalence of Lifetime Psychiatric Disorders Among Black, Hispanic, and Asian Adults in the U.S." *Journal of Psychiatric Research*, January 2013. 47(1): 56–63.

11 A. L. Pieterse et al., "Perceived Racism and Mental Health Among Black American Adults: A Meta-Analytic Review." *Journal of Counseling Psychology*, 2012. 59(1): 1–9.

12 S. E. Carter et al., "The Effect of Early Discrimination on Accelerated Aging Among African Americans." *Health Psychology*, 2019. 38(11): 1010–1013.

13 "NIH Offers New Comprehensive Guide to Healthy Sleep." National Institutes of Health, News Releases, March 23, 2006. https://www.nih.gov/news-events/news-releases/nih -offers-new-comprehensive-guide-healthy-sleep.

14 A. S. Felix et al., "Stress, Resilience, and Cardiovascular Disease Risk Among Black Women." *Circulation: Cardiovascular Quality and Outcomes*, 2019. 12(4): e005284.

15 Table 15, "Life expectancy at birth, at age 65, and at age 75, by sex, race, and Hispanic origin: United States, selected years 1900–2015." National Center for Health Statistics, Centers for Disease Control and Prevention. https://www.cdc.gov /nchs/hus/contents2016.htm#015.

16 "Any Anxiety Disorder." National Institute of Mental Health, Mental Health Information, Statistics, last updated November 2017. https://www.nimh.nih.gov/health/statistics/any -anxiety-disorder.shtml.

17 N. N. Watson and C. D. Hunter, "'I Had to Be Strong':

Tensions in the Strong Black Woman Schema." *Journal of Black Psychology*, 2015. 42(5): 424–452.

18 R. L. Collins and L. D. McNair, "Ethnicity in Alcohol Research." National Institutes of Health, National Institute on Alcohol Abuse and Alcoholism.

19 "Drinking Levels Defined." National Institute on Alcohol Abuse and Alcoholism. https://www.niaaa.nih.gov/alcohol -health/overview-alcohol-consumption/moderate-binge -drinking.

20 E. F. Harrington, J. H. Crowther, and J. C. Shipherd, "Trauma, Binge Eating, and the 'Strong Black Woman.'" *Journal of Consulting and Clinical Psychology*, 2010. 78(4): 469–479.

21 "Obesity and African Americans." US Department of Health and Human Services, Office of Minority Health, last modified March 26, 2020. https://minorityhealth.hhs.gov/omh /browse.aspx?lvl=4&lvlid=25.

22 J. S. Jackson, K. M. Knight, and J. A. Rafferty, "Race and Unhealthy Behaviors: Chronic Stress, the HPA Axis, and Physical and Mental Health Disparities over the Life Course." *American Journal of Public Health*, 2010. 100(5): 933–939.

23 *Stress in America Report*. American Psychological Association, November 9, 2010. https://www.apa.org/news/press /releases/stress/2010/national-report.pdf.

24 A. T. Geronimus et al., "'Weathering' and Age Patterns of Allostatic Load Scores Among Blacks and Whites in the United States." *American Journal of Public Health*, 2006. 96(5): 826–833.

THREE. Intergenerational Trauma

1 C. E. Sartor et al., "Common Heritable Contributions to Low-Risk Trauma, High-Risk Trauma, Posttraumatic Stress Disorder, and Major Depression." *Archives of General Psychiatry*, 2012. 69(3): 293–299.

2 Douglas F. Levinson and Walter E. Nichols, "Major Depression and Genetics." Stanford Medicine, Genetics of Brain Function. https://med.stanford.edu/depressiongenetics/mdd andgenes.html; Jessica Maples-Keller and Vasiliki Michopoulos, "Anxiety Causes and Risk Factors." What Is Anxiety? Anxiety.org. https://www.anxiety.org/what-is-anxiety#:~:text =Genetic%20risk%20factors%20have%20been,risk%20 for%20an%20anxiety%20disorder.

3 "Post-Traumatic Stress Disorder (PTSD)." National Institute of Mental Health, Mental Health Information, Statistics, last updated November 2017. https://www.nimh.nih.gov /health/statistics/post-traumatic-stress-disorder-ptsd.shtml.

4 A. L. Roberts et al., "Race/Ethnic Differences in Exposure to Traumatic Events, Development of Post-Traumatic Stress Disorder, and Treatment-Seeking for Post-Traumatic Stress Disorder in the United States." *Psychological Medicine*, 2011. 41(1): 71–83.

5 "PTSD Facts and Statistics." The Recovery Village, updated September 17, 2020. https://www.therecoveryvillage.com /mental-health/ptsd/related/ptsd-statistics/#:~:text=70%20 percent%20of%20adults%20experience,traumatic%20 event%20will%20develop%20PTSD.

6 Deborah Smith, "Angry Thoughts, At-Risk Hearts." *Monitor on Psychology*, 2003. 34(3): 46. https://www.apa.org/monitor /mar03/angrythoughts.

7   M. L. Slepian, J. S. Chun, and M. F. Mason, "The Experience of Secrecy." *Journal of Personality and Social Psychology*, 2017. 113(1): 1–33.

FOUR. Loss of Innocence

1   *Fourth National Incidence Study of Child Abuse and Neglect (NIS-4): Report to Congress.* US Department of Health and Human Services, Administration for Children and Families, Office of Planning, Research and Evaluation, January 15, 2010; last reviewed December 6, 2018. https://www.acf .hhs.gov/opre/report/fourth-national-incidence-study-child -abuse-and-neglect-nis-4-report-congress.

2   "Child Sexual Abuse Statistics: The Issue of Sexual Abuse." Darkness to Light, 2017. https://www.d2l.org/wp-content /uploads/2017/01/all_statistics_20150619.pdf.

3   "Child Sexual Abuse Statistics: Risk Factors." Darkness to Light, 2017. https://www.d2l.org/wp-content/uploads/2017 /01/Statistics_4_Risk_Factors.pdf.

4   "The Evidence Base: Child Maltreatment Risk Factors." Child and Family Research Partnership, University of Texas at Austin, LBJ School of Public Affairs. https://childandfamilyresearch. utexas.edu/evidence-base-child-maltreatment-risk-factors.

5   "The Evidence Base."

6   Rebecca Epstein, Jamilia J. Blake, and Thalia Gonzalez, *Girlhood Interrupted: The Erasure of Black Girls' Childhood.* Center on Poverty and Inequality, Georgetown Law Center, June 27, 2017. https://www.law.georgetown.edu/poverty -inequality-center/wp-content/uploads/sites/14/2017/08 /girlhood-interrupted.pdf.

7   Jamila Blake and Rebecca Epstein, *Listening to Black Women*

and Girls, Lived Experiences of Adultification Bias. Center on Poverty and Inequality, Georgetown Law Center, 2019. https://genderjusticeandopportunity.georgetown.edu/wp -content/uploads/2020/06/Listening-to-Black-Women -and-Girls.pdf.

8 John Sciamanna, "Child Maltreatment Report Released Includes Increased Numbers." Child Welfare League of America, 2014, https://www.cwla.org/child-maltreatment -report-released-includes-increased-numbers/.

9 Jim DeRogatis, "Inside the Pied Piper of R&B's 'Cult.'" Buzz Feed.news, July 17, 2017. https://www.buzzfeednews.com /article/jimderogatis/parents-told-police-r-kelly-is-keeping -women-in-a-cult#.umLpRYlMDl.

10 John Eligon, "Meet the Woman Asking R. Kelly's Accusers to Come Forward." *New York Times*, January 25, 2019. https://www.nytimes.com/2019/01/25/us/r-kelly-kim-foxx -surviving-documentary.html.

11 Amy Rynell, Katie Buitrago, and Samantha Tuttle, "Cycle of Risk: The Intersection of Poverty, Violence and Trauma, Report on Illinois Poverty." Social Impact Research Center, Heartland Alliance, Ending Poverty, March 15, 2017. https:// socialimpactresearchcenter.issuelab.org/resource/cycle-of -risk-the-intersection-of-poverty-violence-and-trauma-2.html.

12 Jaqueline L. Stock, Debra K. Boyer, and Frederick A. Connell, "Adolescent Pregnancy and Sexual Risk-Taking Among Sexually Abused Girls." *Family Planning Perspectives*, September /October 1997. 29(5): https://doi.org/10.1363/2920097.

13 "How Can I Protect My Child from Sexual Assault?" Rape, Abuse & Incest National Network, n.d. https://www.rainn .org/articles/how-can-i-protect-my-child-sexual-assault.

FIVE. Relationship Baggage

1   "Social Isolation, Loneliness in Older People Pose Health
    Risks." National Institute on Aging, US Department of Health
    and Human Services, April 23, 2019. https://www.nia.nih
    .gov/news/social-isolation-loneliness-older-people-pose-health
    -risks#:~:text=Health%20effects%20of%20social%20isola
    tion,Alzheimer's%20disease%2C%20and%20even%20death.

SIX. I Can Do Bad All by Myself

1   "Preventing Intimate Partner Violence." Violence Prevention,
    Centers for Disease Control and Prevention, last reviewed
    October 29, 2020. https://www.cdc.gov/violenceprevention
    /intimatepartnerviolence/fastfact.html.

2   US Preventive Services Task Force et al., "Screening for Inti-
    mate Partner Violence, Elder Abuse, and Abuse of Vulnerable
    Adults: US Preventive Services Task Force Final Recommen-
    dation Statement." *JAMA,* 2018. 320(16): 1678–1687. doi:
    10.1001/jama.2018.14741.

3   L. Elliott, "Barriers to Screening for Domestic Violence."
    Journal of General Internal Medicine, 2002. 17(2): 112–116.

4   L. B. Meredith Colias-Pete, Ese Olumhense, and Anna Spo-
    erre, "Slain Chicago Doctor Broke Off Engagement with Her
    Killer Weeks Before Deadly Mercy Hospital Shooting." *Chi-
    cago Tribune,* November 21, 2018.

5   E. Petrosky et al., "Racial and Ethnic Differences in Homi-
    cides of Adult Women and the Role of Intimate Partner
    Violence—United States, 2003–2014." *Morbidity and Mor-
    tality Weekly Report,* Centers for Disease Control and Preven-
    tion, July 21, 2017. https://www.cdc.gov/mmwr/volumes
    /66/wr/mm6628a1.htm.

6   "50 Obstacles to Leaving." National Domestic Violence Hot-line. https://www.thehotline.org/resources/50-obstacles-to -leaving/.

7   "M8: Wise Mind." Dialectical Behavior Therapy, n.d. https:// dialecticalbehaviortherapy.com/mindfulness/wise-mind/.

SEVEN. Suffering of the Womb

1   D. E. Dailey et al., "An Exploration of Lifetime Trauma Exposure in Pregnant Low-Income African American Women." *Maternal and Child Health Journal*, 2011. 15(3): 410–418.

2   S. Mukherjee et al., "Risk of Miscarriage Among Black Women and White Women in a U.S. Prospective Cohort Study." *American Journal of Epidemiology*, 2013. 177(11): 1271–1278; M. Willinger, C. W. Ko, and U. M. Reddy, "Racial Disparities in Stillbirth Risk Across Gestation in the United States." *American Journal of Obstetrics & Gynecology*, 2009. 201(5): 469.e1–469.e8.

3   "Racial and Ethnic Disparities Continue in Pregnancy-Related Deaths: Black, American Indian/Alaska Native Women Most Affected." Centers for Disease Control and Prevention, CDC Newsroom, September 5, 2019. https://www.cdc.gov/media /releases/2019/p0905-racial-ethnic-disparities-pregnancy -deaths.html.

4   K. M. Hoffman et al., "Racial Bias in Pain Assessment and Treatment Recommendations, and False Beliefs About Biological Differences Between Blacks and Whites." *Proceedings of the National Academy of Sciences of the USA*, 2016. 113(16): 4296–4301.

5   H. Hutcherson, "Black Women Are Hit Hardest by Fibroid Tumors." *New York Times,* April 15, 2020; E. A. Stewart et al., "The Burden of Uterine Fibroids for African-American

Women: Results of a National Survey." *Journal of Women's Health*, 2013. 22(10): 807–816.

6   D. Baird and L. A. Wise, "Childhood Abuse and Fibroids." *Epidemiology*, 2011. 22(1): 15–17.

7   Renée Boynton-Jarrett et al., "Abuse in Childhood and Risk of Uterine Leiomyoma: The Role of Emotional Support in Biologic Resilience." *Epidemiology*, 2011. 22(1): 6–14. https://journals.lww.com/epidem/pages/articleviewer.aspx?year=2011&issue=01000&article=00002&type=Fulltext.

8   Jennie G. Noll et al., "Obesity Risk for Female Victims of Childhood Sexual Abuse: A Prospective Study." *Pediatrics*, 2007. 120(1): e61–e67. https://pediatrics.aappublications.org/content/pediatrics/120/1/e61.full.pdf.

9   A. I. Vines, M. Ta, and D. A. Esserman, "The Association Between Self-Reported Major Life Events and the Presence of Uterine Fibroids." *Women's Health Issues*, 2010. 20(4): 294–298.

10   "Hysterectomy in the United States: Background." National Women's Health Network, July 9, 2015. https://nwhn.org/hysterectomy/.

11   K. Hartmann et al., *Management of Uterine Fibroids*. Comparative Effectiveness Review No. 195 (Rockville, MD: Agency for Healthcare Research and Quality, 2017). https://www.ncbi.nlm.nih.gov/books/NBK537742/.

12   T. Russell, "Mortality Rate for Black Babies Is Cut Dramatically When Black Doctors Care for Them After Birth, Researchers Say." *Washington Post*, January 13, 2021.

13   T. Pearlstein et al., "Postpartum Depression." *American Journal of Obstetrics and Gynecology*, 2009. 200(4): 357–364.

14   Elizabeth A. Howell et al., "Racial and Ethnic Differences in Factors Associated with Early Postpartum Depressive

Symptoms." *Obstetrics and Gynecology*, 2005, 105(6): 1442–1450. https://pubmed.ncbi.nlm.nih.gov/15932842/.

15 Committee on Obstetric Practice, "Screening for Perinatal Depression," Committee Opinion No. 757. American College of Obstetricians and Gynecologists, November 2018. https://www.acog.org/clinical/clinical-guidance/committee-opinion/articles/2018/11/screening-for-perinatal-depression.

16 K. B. Kozhimannil et al., "Racial and Ethnic Disparities in Postpartum Depression Care Among Low-Income Women." *Psychiatric Services*, 2011. 62(6): 619–625.

EIGHT. The Maternal Bond

1 "Sexual Revictimization Research Brief." National Sexual Violence Resource Center, 2011. https://www.nsvrc.org/publications/nsvrc-publications-research-briefs/sexual-revictimization.

2 S. Clifford and J. Silver-Greenberg, "Foster Care as Punishment: The New Reality of 'Jane Crow.'" *New York Times*, July 21, 2017.

3 Gail Tittle, Philip Garnier, and John Poertner, "Child Maltreatment in Foster Care: A Study of Retrospective Reporting." University of Illinois at Urbana-Champaign. https://cfrc.illinois.edu/pubs/rp_20010501_ChildMaltreatmentInFosterCareAStudyOfRetrospectiveReporting.pdf.

4 Heather D. Boonstra, "Teen Pregnancy Among Young Women in Foster Care: A Primer." *Guttmacher Policy Review*, 2011. 14(2). https://www.guttmacher.org/gpr/2011/06/teen-pregnancy-among-young-women-foster-care-primer.

5 Elizabeth Wall-Wieler et al., "The Cycle of Child Protection Services Involvement: A Cohort Study of Adolescent Mothers."

Pediatrics, 2018. 141(6). https://pediatrics.aappublications
.org/content/141/6/e20173119.

6 "Title IV-E Prevention Program." US Department of Health
and Human Services, Children's Bureau, March 17, 2021.
https://www.acf.hhs.gov/cb/title-iv-e-prevention-program.

NINE. Daddy Issues

1 J. Martin et al., "Births: Final Data for 2018." *National Vital
Statistics Reports*, Centers for Disease Control and Prevention, November 27, 2019. 68(13). https://www.cdc.gov
/nchs/data/nvsr/nvsr68/nvsr68_13-508.pdf.

2 Hal Arkowitz and Scott O. Lilienfeld, "Is Divorce Bad for
Children?" *SA Mind*, 2013. 24(1): 68–69. https://www
.scientificamerican.com/article/is-divorce-bad-for-children/.

3 Arkowitz and Lilienfeld, "Is Divorce Bad for Children?"

TEN. The Buildup

1 Vinita Mehta, "Growing Up with a Mentally Ill Parent: Six
Core Experiences." *Psychology Today,* September 5, 2017.
https://www.psychologytoday.com/us/blog/head-games
/201709/growing-mentally-ill-parent-6-core-experiences.

2 Jacquelyn Y. Taylor et al., "Classification and Correlates of
Eating Disorders Among Blacks: Findings from the National
Survey of American Life." *Journal of Health Care for the Poor
and Underserved*, 2013. 24(1): 289–310. https://www.ncbi
.nlm.nih.gov/pmc/articles/PMC3564508/.

3 H. W. Neighbors et al., "Race, Ethnicity, and the Use of Services
for Mental Disorders: Results from the National Survey of
American Life." *Archives of General Psychiatry*, 2007. 64(4): 485–
494; "Results from the 2012 National Survey on Drug Use and

Health: Mental Health Findings." US Department of Health and Human Services, Substance Abuse and Mental Health Services Administration, Center for Behavioral Health Statistics Quality, September 2013. https://www.samhsa.gov/data/sites /default/files/NSDUHresults2012/NSDUHresults2012.pdf.

4 "1.5 Million Young Adults Do Not Receive Needed Mental Health Services, National Survey on Drug Use Report." Substance Abuse and Mental Health Services Administration: The CBHSQ Report, May 20, 2015. https://www.samhsa .gov/data/report/15-million-young-adults-do-not-receive -needed-mental-health-services.

5 R. R. Cabral and T. B. Smith, "Racial/Ethnic Matching of Clients and Therapists in Mental Health Services: A Meta-Analytic Review of Preferences, Perceptions, and Outcomes." *Journal of Counseling Psychology*, 2011. 58(4): 537–554.

6 Luona Lin, Karen Stamm, and Peggy Christidis, "How Diverse Is the Psychology Workforce?" *Monitor on Psychology*, 2018. 29(2). https://www.apa.org/monitor/2018/02/datapoint.

7 M. Alegría et al., "Inequalities in Use of Specialty Mental Health Services Among Latinos, African Americans, and Non-Latino Whites." *Psychiatric Services*, 2002. 53(12): 1547–1555.

8 "Depression in Adults: Screening." Final Recommendation Statement, US Preventive Services Task Force, January 26, 2016. https://www.uspreventiveservicestaskforce.org/uspstf /document/RecommendationStatementFinal/depression -in-adults-screening.

9 "Mental Health and Substance Abuse Coverage." HealthCare .gov. https://www.healthcare.gov/coverage/mental-health -substance-abuse-coverage/.

10 Ayse Akincigil and Elizabeth B. Matthews, "National Rates

and Patterns of Depression Screening in Primary Care: Results from 2012 and 2013." *Psychiatric Services*, 2017. 68(7): 660–666.

11　J. Unützer and M. Park, "Strategies to Improve the Management of Depression in Primary Care." *Primary Care*, 2012. 39(2): 415–431.

12　L. A. Cooper, "The Acceptability of Treatment for Depression Among African-American, Hispanic, and White Primary Care Patients." *Medical Care*, 2003. 41(4): 479–489; J. L. Givens et al., "Ethnicity and Preferences for Depression Treatment." *General Hospital Psychiatry*, 2007. 29(3): 182–191.

13　M. Alegría et al., "Disparity in Depression Treatment Among Racial and Ethnic Minority Populations in the United States." *Psychiatric Services*, 2008. 59(11): 1264–1272.

14　"The Tuskegee Timeline." Centers for Disease Control and Prevention, March 2, 2020. https://www.cdc.gov/tuskegee /timeline.htm.

15　R. Skloot, *The Immortal Life of Henrietta Lacks* (New York: Crown, 2010).

16　"Incarceration Nation: The United States Leads the World in Incarceration. A New Report Explores Why—and Offers Recommendations for Fixing the System." *Monitor on Psychology*, October 2014.

ELEVEN. The Breakdown

1　C. Carrega, "US Customs and Border Protection Officer Held on $200K Bond for Allegedly Killing Wife on Thanksgiving." ABC News, November 30, 2019. https://abcnews.go.com /US/us-customs-border-protection-officer-held-200k-bond /story?id=67405593.

2   K. O. Conner et al., "Attitudes and Beliefs About Mental Health Among African American Older Adults Suffering from Depression." *Journal of Aging Studies*, 2010. 24(4): 266–277; L. C. Rusch et al., "Depression Stigma in a Predominantly Low Income African American Sample with Elevated Depressive Symptoms." *Journal of Nervous and Mental Disease*, 2008. 196(12): 919–922.

TWELVE. Black People Don't Commit Suicide

1   "Suicide." National Institutes of Mental Health, Mental Health Information, Statistics, last updated January 2021. https://www.nimh.nih.gov/health/statistics/suicide.shtml.

2   "Fast Facts." Suicide Prevention, Centers for Disease Control and Prevention, last reviewed January 21, 2021. https://www.cdc.gov/suicide/facts/index.html.

3   "Suicide Rising Across the US." Centers for Disease Control and Prevention, Vital Signs, last reveiwed June 7, 2018. https://www.cdc.gov/vitalsigns/suicide/index.html.

4   "QuickStats: Age-Adjusted Suicide Rates, by Race/Ethnicity— National Vital Statistics System, United States, 2015–2016." *Morbidity and Mortality Weekly Report*, 2018. 67: 433. https://www.cdc.gov/mmwr/volumes/67/wr/mm6714a6.htm.

5   S. Curtin and H. Hedegaard, "Suicide Rates for Females and Males by Race and Ethnicity: United States, 1999 and 2017." NCHS Health E-Stat 2019, National Center for Health Statistics, Centers for Disease Control and Prevention. https://www.cdc.gov/nchs/data/hestat/suicide/rates_1999_2017.htm.

6   M. A. Lindsey et al., "Trends of Suicidal Behaviors Among High School Students in the United States: 1991–2017." *Pediatrics*, 2019. 144(5): e20191187.

7 J. H. Price and J. Khubchandani, "The Changing Characteristics of African-American Adolescent Suicides, 2001–2017." *Journal of Community Health*, 2019. 44(4): 756–763.

8 "The Relationship Between Bullying and Suicide: What We Know and What It Means for Schools." Centers for Disease Control and Prevention, National Center for Injury Prevention and Control, Division of Violence Prevention, April 2014. https://www.cdc.gov/violenceprevention/pdf/bullying -suicide-translation-final-a.pdf.

9 "African American Suicide Fact Sheet Based on 2014 Data (2016)." American Association of Suicidology. https://www .wellspacehealth.org/wp-content/uploads/2016/10/African -American-Suicide-Fact-Sheet-2016.pdf.

10 R. J. Taylor, L. M. Chatters, and S. Joe, "Religious Involvement and Suicidal Behavior Among African Americans and Black Caribbeans." *Journal of Nervous and Mental Disease*, 2011. 199(7): 478–486.

11 T. J. VanderWeele et al., "Association Between Religious Service Attendance and Lower Suicide Rates Among US Women." *JAMA Psychiatry*, 2016. 73(8): 845–851.

12 Lindsay K. Admon et al., "Trends in Suicidality 1 Year Before and After Birth Among Commercially Insured Child-Bearing Individuals in the United States, 2006–2017." *JAMA Psychiatry*, 2021. 78(2): 171–176. https://jamanetwork.com /journals/jamapsychiatry/article-abstract/2772882?guest AccessKey=a43e83d4-e8a7-4484-98e6-804de93a8236&utm _source=For_The_Media&utm_medium=referral&utm_cam paign=ftm_links&utm_content=tfl&utm_term=111820.

THIRTEEN. Maybe I Should Talk to Someone

1 I. Burnett-Zeigler et al., "A Mindfulness-Based Intervention for Low-Income African American Women with Depressive Symptoms Delivered by an Experienced Instructor Versus a Novice Instructor." *Journal of Alternative and Complementary Medicine*, 2019. 25(7): 699–708.

FOURTEEN. Let Go and Let God

1 L. M. Chatters et al., "Religious Coping Among African Americans, Caribbean Blacks and Non-Hispanic Whites." *Journal of Community Psychology*, 2008. 36(3): 371–386.

2 "A Religious Portrait of African-Americans." Pew Research Center, Religion and Public Life, January 30, 2009. https://www.pewforum.org/2009/01/30/a-religious-portrait-of-african-americans/.

3 K. Sambol-Tosco, "The Slave Experience: Religion." Slavery and the Making of America. https://www.thirteen.org/wnet/slavery/experience/religion/history.html.

4 R. Whitley, "'Thank You God': Religion and Recovery from Dual Diagnosis Among Low-Income African Americans." *Transcultural Psychiatry*, 2012. 49(1): 87–104.

5 K. S. Johnson, K. I. Elbert-Avila, and J. A. Tulsky, "The Influence of Spiritual Beliefs and Practices on the Treatment Preferences of African Americans: A Review of the Literature." *Journal of the American Geriatrics Society*, 2005. 53(4): 711–719.

6 H. W. Neighbors, M. A. Musick, and D. R. Williams, "The African American Minister as a Source of Help for Serious Personal Crises: Bridge or Barrier to Mental Health Care?" *Health Education and Behavior*, 1998. 25(6): 759–777.

7   L. A. Cooper et al., "How Important Is Intrinsic Spirituality in Depression Care? A Comparison of White and African-American Primary Care Patients." *Journal of General Internal Medicine*, 2001. 16(9): 634–638.

8   Amanda T. Woodward et al., "Complementary and Alternative Medicine for Mental Disorders Among African Americans, Black Caribbeans, and Whites." *Psychiatric Services*, 2009. 60(10): 1342–1349.

9   W. Dessio et al., "Religion, Spirituality, and Healthcare Choices of African-American Women: Results of a National Survey." *Ethnicity and Disease*, 2004. 14(2): 189–197.

10 M. N. Wittink et al., "Losing Faith and Using Faith: Older African Americans Discuss Spirituality, Religious Activities, and Depression." *Journal of General Internal Medicine*, 2009. 24(3): 402–407.

11 C. Routledge, "What Prayer Is Good For—and the Evidence for It." *National Review*, April 9, 2018.

FIFTEEN. Self-Care Is Not Selfish

1   "How Much Physical Activity Do Adults Need?" Physical Activity, Centers for Disease Control and Prevention, last reviewed October 7, 2020. https://www.cdc.gov/physicalactivity/basics/adults/index.htm.

SIXTEEN. Joy Comes in the Morning

1   Dorairaj Prabhakaran and Ambalam M. Chandrasekaran, "Yoga for the Prevention of Cardiovascular Disease." *Nature Reviews Cardiology*, 2020. 17: 536–537. https://www.nature.com/articles/s41569-020-0412-x.

About the Author

DR. INGER BURNETT-ZEIGLER is a clinical psychologist and associate professor in the Department of Psychiatry and Behavioral Sciences, Feinberg School of Medicine, at Northwestern University. She has more than fifteen years of experience providing psychological interventions to help clients experiencing depression, anxiety, traumatic stress, and relationship strain. Her scholarly work focuses on the role of social determinants of health on disparities in mental illness and treatment, particularly in the Black community. Dr. Burnett-Zeigler is a fierce advocate for eliminating mental illness stigma and assuring that all individuals have access to high-quality, evidence-based mental health care. Her writing has appeared in the *New York Times*, *The Hill*, and the *Chicago Tribune*. She was born and raised in Chicago, where she currently lives.